ASKING AND GIVING

A Report on Hospital Philanthropy

Robert M. Cunningham Jr.

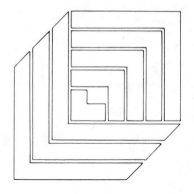

American Hospital Association
840 North Lake Shore Drive
Chicago, Illinois 60611

Library of Congress Cataloging in Publication Data

Cunningham, Robert Maris, 1909-
   Asking and giving.

   "AHA catalog no. 1030."
   Includes bibliographical references and index.
   1. Hospitals—Endowments.   2. Hospitals—
Finance.   3. Fund raising.   4. Public relations—
Hospitals.   5. Hospitals—United States—Endowments.
I. Title. [DNLM: 1. Financial management.
2. Hospital administration—United States. WX157.3
C973a]
RA971.3.C86   362.1'1   79-28315
ISBN 0-87258-300-7

AHA catalog no. 1030
© 1980 by the
American Hospital Association
840 North Lake Shore Drive
Chicago, Illinois 60611

The views expressed in this book are those of the author.

Contents

Preface

The first boss I ever had, outside of caddymasters and drugstore managers during vacations, was a fund raiser who had finished a building campaign for a Chicago hospital and had been retained to do the same thing for a small private college. It seemed a bizarre thing for me to be doing, but my father had a close friend who was a trustee of the college, and in those days of deepening depression the goal was gainful employment, not career strategy. My classmates and I had quickly discovered that wherever we applied for jobs, they had just laid off 40 or 50 of their best people. We took what we could get.

As it turned out, I was one of the lucky ones. The job lasted two years, and we spent most of the time organizing the trustees and faculty to get money from the alumni and the alumni to get it from each other. The depression kept getting worse, and the right time—or anything but an obviously disastrous time—for a public campaign never did come, and the fund raiser I worked for spent most of the time when he wasn't meeting with alumni telling the trustees how they ought to reorganize the college. When they couldn't afford him any longer, we were both out of jobs. He became a management consultant and made a fortune, and I went to work in a gas station. It was that kind of time.

Later, largely on the basis of my knowledge of fund-raising techniques, which exceeded my baby-sister's, but not by much, I got a job at a hospital that was beginning to flex its biceps preparatory to undertaking an expansion program. My duties included interviewing trustees and staff members as part of the process of accumulating a stockpile of needs for added space and new facilities. I was long gone before any intensive capital fund raising was initiated, but I was involved in the activities that produced annual contributions to the free care fund, as it was called, and I spent a lot of time at trustee meetings where prospective donors were evaluated. My other tasks were concerned with the institution's publicity and publication requirements. Those were still depression years, and, looking back, I estimate that I may have been the only hospital public relations person in existence then. But I wasn't the first. The first one was St. Luke. We don't know much about his methods, but we all know what a great job he did for the Good Samaritan.

Until recently, the only other opportunities I've had to observe the development species in its native habitat came about because I had two friends who both became institutional development officers, though that isn't what they were called. One was assistant to the president of a university, and the other was administrator of a small but prestigious hospital that was run by the chief of surgery. Actually, my two friends had identical jobs. They were both fund raisers, and they were very good at it. One had retired early from a family business that bored him, and the other had run out of family money and needed the job. Both were well connected, as we say. They knew where the money was and could call it by its first name. They invited the right doctor on the hospital staff or the right scientist on the university faculty to lunch with the right money. They had the natural grace to make such occasions work, and with astonishing regularity the money ended up on the other side of the table. Both of them loved the institutions they worked for, and loved their work, and among all the fund raisers I've talked to since then, I haven't discovered a better formula for success.

What I have discovered mainly is that it's a lot more complicated than that now. For one thing, nobody knows where all the money is anymore. Finding it isn't easy; there are many more competing demands—on the money, on the doctors and scientists, and on the development and fund-raising people, who now have to use computers to produce the records and reports my friends used to carry around in their heads or on cards in their pockets.

I found all this out after I had lightheartedly agreed to undertake the present exercise, thinking it would be a matter of looking up and interviewing a few of the people who are now doing what my friends used to do a generation ago, persuading them to let me sit in on a few of their cozy little luncheons, and reporting how it is done. I discovered right away that today's methods are necessarily different. But the process is essentially the same; it's still a matter of getting the donor, or sometimes the donor's representative, face to face with the doctor or scientist for whose work support is needed, or with the appropriate surrogates who are hospital administrators or trustees or consultants or volunteers. And again, if the process has been properly prepared and conducted, and the moon is in the right quarter, the money is likely to move.

But I hadn't talked to very many of the principals or surrogates on either side of the transaction before I discovered something else: The work my friends were doing back there in those simpler times was a lot harder than it looked. It had always seemed so relaxed and pleasant, as much pastime as vocation. But I understand now that they had to know a whole host of things: about donors and about their institutions and the people who worked in them. And I also now understand that those seemingly casual luncheons were probably as carefully planned and prepared, and possibly rehearsed, as the most formidable foundation conferences are. I expect it *was* easier to raise money for hospitals and universities a generation ago than it is today, but not that much easier.

Another thing that I have found as I have been making my way around among the fund raisers and development people off and on during the past two years is that they are extraordinarily earnest about what they are doing. My friends who were their professional predecessors loved their institutions and their work, and so do today's torch bearers. I had thought that the fund-raising consultant who spends his life skipping from hospital to college to church to YMCA must become a cynical fellow who has seen everything and considers one scam about like another, but unless I happened on only the exceptions—and my method was random, if not wild—I found precisely the contrary to be the case. However modest the institution, its continued and improved function is as the fate of nations. When you stop to think about it for a minute, how could it be otherwise? The consultant is a latter-day nomad whose habitat is the suitcase, and who would live that way if he didn't think it was essential to the survival of the society? Unlike the economic circumstance that got me into the fund-raising business in 1931, today's economy provides other ways of making a living.

The institutional development officer is more of the same, probably with an added attachment, if anything, for the insitution and its mission. There is a certain amount of career job-hopping among the younger members of the calling, to be sure, but no more than there is among young bankers or hospital administrators, and a whole lot less than among young advertising agency executives, who share many of the same talents and are about as constant as a firefly.

As I have reported here, the development officer is essentially an optimistic organism. As a rational being, he has to be nervous about the future and worried about the volatility of the income tax, the whimsy of the bureaucrat, and the eccentricities the Congress is capable of accommodating. But he has faith that these will all be ironed out in time and that he is helping to get the job done, all the while contributing to the better world his institution is creating. It is not all pure Pangloss, however, because development people are an informed and intelligent lot, and neither is it laid on or put on like a uniform that goes with the job, although it is certainly true that a fund raiser or development officer with a misanthropic outlook would be something like a coloratura with laryngitis.

The development view of the world is not widely shared among hospital administrators, whose hypothesis today is more likely to be that the world is going to hell and hospitals are being pushed into leading the way. Obviously, administrators come in all sizes and shapes, as well as all casts of mind. Not all of them are despairing, and those who are will tell you that if you think things are going to get better it is only because you do not understand the problem, and they could be right. But it has seemed to me to be true that it is among the exceptions to the generally cheerless majority that one can find those administrators who are outstanding fund raisers. When this is the case, when the administrator is good at fund raising and knows it and thinks it is important and makes time for it, nobody can do it better. Nobody else knows the institution as he does. It will be noted in this report, too, that some donors are strongly motivated not by the desire to save the world but only by the wish to stave off disaster, and nobody can scare them into giving the way the administrator can.

Of course, generalizations such as these are risky, and probably foolish, since I have talked only to handfuls out of thousands. But my impression in pursuing the handfuls is that trustees are usually better askers than administrators, partly because most of them are givers themselves and partly because they are likely to know the donors better, but also partly because they are less harassed and depressed about the hospital and can see the bright vision of the future as well as the shape of next week's impending calamity. And the rare physician who can, and is willing to, look away from his patients and his oscillographs long enough to meet with prospective donors can often be the best money raiser of all. His view of the world doesn't matter one way or the other, because it is his patients and his oscillographs that absorb the donor's interest, as they do his. The trustees and administrators and development officers who can convince a few of their physicians that it isn't just the hospital but the whole practice of medicine whose future may be secured by the incomes and estates and trust funds of the wealthy are going to get their share, no matter who is doing the work. And the physicians who practice among the minks and Mercedes can be the hospital's keenest bird-dogs, as long as the development officer has sense enough to refer to that function in somewhat more elevated terms.

That all these and other tricks and trends of the asking business are reported in the following pages resulted from a feeling the publisher of the American Hospital Association first shared with me nearly three years ago: namely, that the pressures of cost containment and certificate of need and quality assurance and

malpractice and political action, among others, had not only turned attention away from philanthropy as a source of hospital
capital and revenue but had more or less convinced a lot of
hospital people that it wouldn't remain a source of hospital capital
and revenue long enough to make it worth worrying about—a conclusion that would obviously hasten the result they foresaw.
Maybe it was time to look around and see what was really happen-
ing and let people know, the publisher suggested.

It took me an unconscionably long time to start looking around,
and what with other errands having to do for the most part with
cost containment and certificate of need and quality assurance and
malpractice and political action, it has taken even longer for me to
put this report together, random and modest as it may be. But it
didn't take that long for me to become certain that the publisher
was at least half right. A lot of hospital people have turned away
from philanthropy and are half-baked in their approach to it, and
thus helping to make it a forgotten art. But a lot more are working
at it more intensively, and more intelligently, than they have ever
done before. They see contributed capital and revenues as rapidly
becoming the only money they have that they can spend the way
they want to, and they are thus helping to keep what we still have
of philanthropy as an art to be cherished and nourished. I hope
that my look around, as reported here, may help persuade more of
the former to join the latter, and show them how.

CHAPTER 1

Giving

Most gifted fund raisers, whether they are university presidents, physicians, hospital administrators or trustees, priests, politicians, or institutional development officers or consultants, believe they know why people give them money for their causes and institutions. The director of a children's hospital may tell you that it's because the donor's heart goes out to the suffering children and he can't resist doing his part to make sure they get the help they need. The university president or development executive may liken the lure of advancing knowledge to the fascination for the unknown that drove Marco Polo halfway around the world centuries ago. The fund-raising professional will point to the universal human need for recognition, as demonstrated by the lasting presence of the memorial plaque. The priest or nun or minister will quote scripture to prove that philanthropists are simply responding to God's will. One consultant will acknowledge that some emotional appeal is always present and then explain that the clincher, in any case, is likely to be a critical tax or estate advantage that makes the gift a sound investment, and another will insist that the basic drive is selfish, actually, because the giver is seeking ego satisfaction in some way.

They are all right. Obviously, there isn't any one reason people give; motivation for giving, as for most behavior, is complex. But there are some recognizable common factors among the reasons people give to particular institutions or causes. "Part of it is a strong feeling and commitment to the institution itself, but wrapped up in that is the absolute faith and belief in the person who heads the institution," said Jerold Panas, a consultant who manages capital fund campaigns for hospitals, colleges, churches, and YMCAs.

As an example, Panas described an orphanage in Cuernavaca, Mexico, for which his firm has conducted successful fund drives. "People feel sorry for orphans, and that's part of it," he said. "But there are orphans all over the world, and they don't have to give money to this one, even if they may have visited Cuernavaca. They give because of the magnetism of Father Wassan, the priest who heads the institution. He has a way of getting under their skin and inspires an absolute belief in what he's doing. I've watched him repeatedly, and he's simply not an effective salesman. He doesn't do anything right. He isn't even especially articulate. But somehow there is a kind of concentration on his part; nothing else interferes with his direct line to another person, and he is able to communicate what he is doing and communicate the love between him and his children. It's not eloquent, but it always gets to the person."[1]

At the Scripps Clinic and Research Foundation in La Jolla, California, it was a physician on the staff who was the chief executive officer and was responsible for the most successful fundraising efforts, Panas related. "He was a masterful strategist, and there wasn't anything left to chance when he was approaching somebody for a major gift," Panas said of the doctor with the magic touch. "He had thought it all out in advance and knew where he was going. But most of all, it was always a person who was related to him in some way; the largest gifts came from people who were devoted to him. They weren't always his patients, but they believed in him, and they believed in the work he was doing."

In some cases, the critical emotional factor can be a feeling for the institution itself, rather than for a person connected with it, Panas allowed. "But the key to giving is emotion, and the emotion can be from several directions. I don't think people give for tax reasons, although if there's an advantage, that's fine. I don't think they give logically. Not many people make a list of a half dozen institutions that are asking them for gifts and logically weigh the pros and cons of each institution. In the case of most people there's a gut feeling that 'I love this place, and I love what they are trying to do. It's exciting, and it appeals to me.' I'm convinced that's why people give.''

Another talented fund raiser, Chase N. Peterson, M.D., former vice-president for development of Harvard University, added another common dimension of emotional involvement: participation. "The whole world of philanthropy means involvement, and involvement means asking people to come in and give their opinions," Peterson said. It isn't an easy thing to do, he added. "If any of us expect to live buoyed up by community support, this has to be achieved at some price of so-called efficiency. We're offering these potential donors involvement in something larger than themselves. We're in the pathways whereby people can exercise vital power in some kind of apparatus or system that has scope. The love of an institution, the love of the healing process, the love of the educational process, love of the mind. It seems to me that we are offering much more than we're getting," he told a group of hospital development officers. "You've all had the experience of having your most generous donor come up and say, 'Thank you for these years when I've been deeply involved in the affairs of this institution. You've allowed me to do something very special in my lifetime.''[2]

Peterson also touched on the added stimulus to generosity provided by recognition. He related an anecdote about Abram Sacher, Ph.D., the first chancellor of Brandeis University, whose success in attracting support for his institution is legendary among practitioners of the art: "The story goes that he had attended a performance in the Brandeis theater, which had been the gift of a generous donor, five or ten years after the gift was given, and then he had just dropped a handwritten note to the donor, taking no more than a minute to write. 'Dear Mr. X,' the note said, 'I just attended a performance of Hamlet in your theater. I wanted you to know that the theater was packed. The pleasure your theater brought to that campus community was enormous, and I want to thank you again.' Well, now, Dr. Sacher was wise enough to know that there was probably something prospectively good about that letter. But he was also wise enough to know that this is part of the web of human society that ought to be fun to do. He did it, and he got a million dollars by return mail. You can interpret that any way you want to, but I can't think of anything more rewarding than picking out those occasions when you can thank someone long after you have to. The first thank-you doesn't do any good, because that is expected and perfunctory and no matter what you say it's pretty much discounted. It's the unnecessary thing that is remembered."

Because memorial plaques have become commonplace as a form of recognition, they might be put down as expected and perfunctory, but that isn't the way most fund raisers or philanthropists regard them. "In your visit to Baylor you noticed innumerable plaques and in some instances oil paintings, and we also have buildings that have been named for major donors," Boone Powell, chairman of the executive committee of Baylor University Medical Center, said recently in a letter to a friend. Powell has been associated with Baylor for 25 years and has been chiefly responsible in that time for the growth of the medical center plant from $5 million to more than $100 million, a large part of which has been contributed by philanthropists—and not a dollar of which has come from tax sources. The visitor had spent a day with Powell and A. Webb Roberts, a Dallas millionaire who had recently given the medical center $1 million to endow a continuing education center. Conversations with Roberts and Powell indicated that they had known each other for years and had often discussed Roberts' interest in education as a benefactor and trustee of Dallas Baptist College. Together, they had developed the concept of the Webb Roberts Continuing Education Center for Baylor. Roberts had obviously enjoyed and benefited from his involvement with the medical center, and at the time the endowment was announced Powell had planned an inauguration program titled "Great Ideas in Surgery," with the nationally known surgical specialists as participants. Later, the surgical lectures were published in a commemorative volume. The recognition programs also included a plaque and portrait of Roberts, which are on display at the center.

Another aspect of donor recognition that is often criticized by educators but that Powell, along with many others, considers suitable and effective, is the awarding of honorary degrees. "Of course, one does not buy a degree with a gift," Powell said. "But in the case of someone like Webb Roberts the cumulative good deeds and outstanding civic service over a long period of years earn recognition of this type. Webb was awarded an honorary doctor of laws degree by Dallas Baptist College not only for his service to the college but for his other good works over a long period. In my opinion, this type of recognition is valuable and justified."[3]

The honorary degree and the portrait may be regarded as special flourishes for special cases, but the bronze plaque is the standard of philanthropic recognition, as the walls and halls of hospitals and colleges all over the country plainly testify. There are no precise criteria in square inches of plaque per thousand dollars of gift, perhaps, but every institution has its hierarchy of values: so much for the room, and so much more for the floor, wing, pavilion, or building. There is no guarantee to the donor or the family that the plaque will endure forever, to be sure. But any institution faces a logistics problem, and perhaps a moral problem as well, when an old, plaque-ridden building has to be vacated or torn down, sacrificed to the demands of expansion and progress. More often than not, the places that were suitable for the old plaques do not exist in the new environment, and in any case the place of honor at the main entrance that commemorated the major donor of the old building either has to be given over to the major donor to the new building or used for some other purpose. In the new capital culture, there are no plaques perpetuating the memory of the bankers who approved the mortgage loans.

When the Monongalia General Hospital vacated the buildings it has occupied for years in the busy center of Morgantown, West Virginia, and moved to a new hilltop site on the outskirts of town, members of Morgantown families whose fathers and grandfathers had been benefactors of the hospital were upset. "The family whose plaque was on Room 128 in the old building thought the plaque should be put up at Room 128 in the new building," said David Woodrum, the administrator, who was prepared to cope with the inevitable problems of moving a hospital, which are numbered in millions, but was baffled by this one. The solution worked out by Woodrum and others when they moved into the new hospital in 1978 must be unique. From the rugged mountains surrounding Morgantown they imported a huge granite boulder, shaped something like the rock of Gibraltar, and installed it on the lawn in front of the hospital entrance. Crowning the boulder is a symbolic bronze cross, recast from all the plaques removed from the old buildings, and on the boulder's sheer face is a new plaque, also recast from the old ones, relating the story of the buildings they honored.[4] As far as anybody knows, the families are all satisfied with this recycled memorial to their generosity.

The testimony of the philanthropist suggests that the most effective recognition of all, however, may come from within. "Most important psychologically is what giving does to the giver," said William Black, chairman of a New York restaurant chain who has given millions to New York medical schools and hospitals and is founder and president of the Parkinson's Disease Foundation. "Wouldn't you be thrilled to feel financially responsible, partly or wholly, for a major breakthrough in the fight against a dread disease? I know the wonderful emotion I would feel if the Parkinson's Disease Foundation finds the cure it seeks while I am still alive. I am thrilled to see my name inscribed on a plaque in the Columbia University Medical Research Center. Who wouldn't be? Doesn't the author feel joy seeing his book in the bookstore window? Doesn't the artist sign his painting out of a feeling of accomplishment? I, too, am quietly happy and deeply thankful that I have been and am able to contribute something to society."[5]

The possibility that some philanthropists may not fully understand why giving makes them happy was raised by Ben Whitaker, a British writer, in a book about foundations. "Some capitalists have a desire to indulge in conspicuous philanthropic expenditure, in the same way as our ancestors used to sacrifice valued animals to thank the gods," Whitaker wrote. "The study of the altruistic expression of feelings has been relatively neglected, but the view of some psychologists is that altruism can be a way of satisfying one's self-love by means of the lives of other people, while avoiding involvement in direct human relationships. Just as the compulsion to accumulate unnecessary wealth can denote a lack of confidence and need to seek recognition by demonstrating, literally, the 'goods' of oneself, so altruism—like asceticism or pharisaism— can be a way of trying to purge this aggressive greed of which a person may feel ashamed. But other psychologists have interpreted altruism as not only a drive to make some reparation, but also as an attempt to spread guilt feelings about gains which are unearned or the product of exploitation."[6] In a definition of philanthropy, a cynical Washington newsman said it this way: "It is people getting credit for giving back what their ancestors should never have taken in the first place." Happily, there are also psychologists who point out that normal donors may simply identify with their bene- ficiaries and so share the satisfaction they are giving.

The combination of philosophic, social, and personal reasons for giving is most often in evidence when philanthropists are will- ing to talk about their benefactions, which many prefer not to do. When Dr. and Mrs. Malcolm Coutts gave the Donald M. Sharp Memorial Hospital in San Diego a trust fund of $1.2 million, Dr. Coutts said they hoped to benefit the people of San Diego through their gift to the hospital's orthopedic-neurologic pavilion. Also, "We wanted to give back to the Sharp Hospital what Sharp Hospital has given us," said Dr. Coutts, who has been a member of the staff for many years. But an additional motive for the gift, he explained, was the desire "to substitute our own will for the hand of government bueaucracy in the disposal of the principal amount of our estate." Their five children would not inherit the principal sum of the estate, diminished by taxes, he said, but they would inherit the income from the undiminished trust estate for as long as they lived.

"It is the political will of our people that large estates cannot be inherited," Dr. Coutts continued. "On the other hand, principal sums left to such charities are not taxed. Our government forgoes its taxes when the principal sum of a bequest goes to a recipient that is nonprofit and engages in approved charitable endeavors. We feel that we should like to designate the uses to which the resources of our estate should be put eventually, rather than have them greatly diminished by taxes, filtered through the government bureaucracy, then distributed to many uses—some of them good, some ineffectual. We should like our estate to be used for the benefit of the people of San Diego. It is in the compassionate care of the sick, the wounded, and the worried that our society displays its most admirable quality, which is mercy, 'where earthly power doth then show likest God's.' "[7]

A distinctive feeling and philosophic conviction have also guided the philanthropies of Foster G. McGaw, the still active founder, honorary chairman, and director of the American Hospital Supply Corporation, who told a visitor not long after his 80th birthday that he had given away approximately $60 million, although an American Hospital Supply executive estimated that the total of McGaw's benefactions over the years might readily aggregate twice that amount, measured in today's dollars. Whatever the total, in most of McGaw's gifts to universities, colleges, and medical centers, three lines of thought are evident: the desire to honor his mother and father; the belief that "God has been so generous with me that I owe Him all this, and it's got to go back to help people," as he told the visitor; and the strong conviction that the substitution of government for private support of institutions leads to mediocrity in a society that depends for its survival and well-being on excellence.

McGaw has been a generous supporter of, among other institutions, Northwestern University and its McGaw Medical Center, the Loyola University Medical Center and its Foster G. McGaw Hospital, and the McCormick Theological Seminary, all in or near Chicago; the American College of Hospital Administrators; and the Association of University Programs in Health Administration. At the time of this visit, he and Mrs. McGaw had just given at least $1 million each to 32 small colleges, to be used for whatever purposes their trustees and administrators should choose. "We've picked out schools that we believe do several things," he explained. "First, they represent Christian ethics. They represent the moralities that we believe in, and then most of them are dedicated to the principle of self help. There are exceptions, but in most cases these colleges won't take students who don't work to pay for their own education. This makes the education so much more valuable, and these are the kinds of people we have tried to support."[8]

McGaw's first large gift to Northwestern University came about because the university had invited the World Council of Churches to meet in Evanston, Illinois, where the university campus is located, and didn't have any place large enough to accommodate the meeting. A fund-raising drive was undertaken, and McGaw's $400,000 donation ensured the success of the enterprise. McGaw Hall became a center for university athletic, cultural, and community affairs. At McCormick Seminary, a Presbyterian institution, McGaw endowed professorships honoring his father, a Presbyterian minister, and an uncle who was a missionary in India. He also gave $1 million for the library at the seminary, which is representative of the strong religious motivation that is characteristic of McGaw's philanthropies. But the religious feeling isn't sectarian. He offered to bet the president of Loyola University that his gifts to the medical center there were more than all Presbyterians put together had given Catholic institutions. "They've got some wonderful people out there," he said of Loyola. "They're alert, intelligent, and well trained, and I think there isn't a medical center in this country that is any better than they are. This is what got me interested, and this is why I've supported them."

McGaw's strong feelings for his father, mother, and uncle are examples of another powerful motivating force in philanthropy. More often than not, the memorial plaque honors not the donor, but a parent, child, or some other person for whom the donor has had a deep emotional attachment. Thus a trustee of a midwestern hospital who has been a generous donor to the institution over the years explained that his attachment was inherited. "My mother and father made a major gift for one of the buildings when I was growing up," he explained. "I'm not sure I understood it then, but I did later as their interest in the hospital, and their gifts, continued, and now I've tried to carry on for the family as I can with my own contributions." Such family hierarchies of trusteeship and philanthropy are not uncommon. Fund raisers seek out families with a tradition of giving, knowing that the fact of giving may be taken for granted, and the task here is simply to determine how much, when, and what for—but knowing also that the tradition doesn't always stand up. Some sons and daughters of wealthy families would rather spend, or waste, than give.

Whether it is inherited or acquired, the best donors have what one hospital development officer has called an innate need to give. "They have this charitable bent that has probably been developed over the years," said Eleanor Heldt of Memorial Hospital Medical Center of Long Beach, California. "It might have started with their church, or it might have been the Boy Scouts, the Girl Scouts, or whatever. It's something that has been growing in them for a number of years, and then when you match that up with something else—a particular illness or experience in the hospital with a member of the family, or perhaps a capital gains or estate tax problem—it has a tendency many times to push them over the edge into a charitable contribution, where they might not make that large gift without having developed the habit of giving."⁹

The particular illness or the hospital experience alone may be all it takes in many instances. Families often may want to give tangible expression of their gratitude for the care an institution or a physician has given a loved one. Some physicians are sensitive to these feelings and may suggest that a gift to the hospital or its foundation, or perhaps a special research fund, would be a suitable gesture. Others are reluctant to make any such suggestions themselves but will let an administrator or trustee or development officer know that an approach to the family might be productive. Many doctors won't ever think of it unless they are reminded from time to time that such opportunities exist, and some don't care and wouldn't do it anyway. The most common answer when development people are asked about the role of physicians as participants in fund raising is, "One or two of the doctors on the staff are very good at it, and I wish we could get more of them interested in taking part."

Of all the reasons people are moved or persuaded to give to charitable institutions and causes, the most persuasive is widely believed to be the religious impulse. Nearly all religions foster charity and elevate generosity of spirit. The tithe existed before the tax, and in many societies it is still considered first among all man's obligations. In the United States, nearly half of all private funds given for all causes is for religious purposes. And it is possible that the religious sector of philanthropy may be even greater than that, because the amounts given to religion are only estimates; nobody really knows. According to a recent *Yearbook* of the National Council of Churches, a Protestant organization, its financial data "are only a significant part of total contributions from members of all communions." Sources of data for the Catholic and Jewish faiths, except for funds used to construct facilities, are correspondingly imprecise. Also, in most compilations, funds given to church-related schools, colleges, and hospitals are counted as contributions to education and health, not religion. But it is likely that in most cases religion may have been a motivating factor, and in some cases the most persuasive or perhaps the only reason for giving.

"While it may be straining a definition to describe sectarian fund raising for hospitals, child care centers, and homes for the aged as religious, there is no doubt that loyalty to the various faiths furnishes the emotional stimulus required to make their annual campaigns successful," wrote George C. Kirstein, whose fund-raising experience includes serving on the boards of trustees of two voluntary hospitals, two educational institutions, a foundation, and several other voluntary agencies depending on contributions for support.[10]

Certainly some consideration of religion is discernible in the philanthropies of donors like Foster McGaw, Webb Roberts, and Malcolm Coutts, and in many cases of giving to hospitals the religious motivation is obviously central. A form of religious philanthropy of a somewhat variant species is the central impelling force in a controversial new medical center now under construction in Tulsa, Oklahoma. According to the Tulsa Hospital Council and the Oklahoma Health Systems Agency, the area already has more hospital beds than it needs. But these professional and planning groups were no match for the political power of an aroused body of believers, and the State Health Planning Commission overrode the planners and gave its approval to the City of Faith Medical Center of Oral Roberts University. Contributions for the center reportedly amounting to $30 or $40 million were received in the first year following announcement of the project, and Oral Roberts, founder and head of the university, the City of Faith Medical Center, and the Oral Roberts Evangelistic Association (the parent organization of these and other enterprises), is confi-

dent that the $150 million or so required to complete the center will
flow in from millions of Oral Roberts "partners," as they are
called, in response to his televised appeals for support.

According to Roberts, God asked him to build the City of Faith,
which he says will become a worldwide referral center providing
medical services for followers of his fundamentalist faith. It
wasn't just a casual conversation, either, Roberts told a newpaper
reporter in an interview about the university and the center. God
appeared before him shortly after his daughter died in 1977,
Roberts related, and when he asked how he could build such a
costly institution, God said, "You can't. I will build it through
you, and I want it built debt free."[11] It will be.

Like many of its kind, the Oral Roberts movement partakes of
both religion and ideology, and ideologies of all kinds are themselves a powerful force in philanthropy. Thus many foundations
are devoted solely to the advancement of particular modes of
thought, and philanthropists like McGaw, Webb Roberts, and
Coutts were plainly motivated in part by the desire to help ensure
that private rather than government resources, and hence decisions, shall prevail in the health care system.

The same ideology was a compelling factor in the mind of
William Black, who gave Columbia University $5 million for a
medical research center. "Private initiative has helped create great
centers of learning that have led the fight against disease," he said.
"Private initiative has given the world's highest standard of living
to most of our people. And yet, we have not eliminated poverty or
disease. Unless those of us who have profited so much from a free
society are willing and able to wipe out its malignities, then men of
extreme convictions will do it for us—at our expense. Philanthropists play a crucial role in our society. If they forget that essen-
tials come first, then philanthropists, who owe their fame and fortune to free enterprise, will be contributing to its deterioration. On
the other hand, they can help speed and perpetuate our country's
unique opportunities for growth if they remember to put first
things first."[12]

In a book about foundations and philanthropy, Washington journalist Joseph C. Goulden reminds us that there are limitations on ideological giving. "What the rich do with their money in private is their own business," he said. "But once they claim the privilege of tax exemption, each of us acquires an interest in the dollars involved, and we deserve to know how and why they are being spent."[13]

CHAPTER 2

Asking and Giving Today

At the time de Tocqueville made his observations of American society and remarked on our extraordinary capacity for organizing voluntary committees and associations to provide resources and services that were considered proper functions of government in most European societies in 1845, our country was near the beginning of a century of expanding industry and corresponding expansion of philanthropy. Men in increasing numbers were making fortunes from a land rich in resources and giving fortunes to found and expand institutions of all kinds. They're still at it, and giving for philanthropic causes is still growing, contrary to what has been a widely held conviction ever since the first federal income tax act was passed in 1913. In that first year, less than 1 percent of the population filed returns, to an accompaniment of gloomy predictions that the new tax would inhibit initiative and stifle private charity.

The prediction became a seeming certainty when the Revenue Act of 1928 raised the surtax rate to 20 percent on net incomes in excess of $100,000, and the number of taxpayers jumped beyond the previous wartime high to 6 percent of the population. Charitable giving reached an all-time high in 1929, however, but thereafter it languished briefly, not because of taxes but because of depression. It's been rising ever since, notwithstanding the setbacks that have accompanied depressions and recessions, bear markets, wars, inflation, and the crotchets of a Congress that has never left off tinkering with taxes and never will.

Total philanthropic giving in the United States reached $6 billion in 1955. It had doubled in the next 10 years, and by 1969 had topped $18 billion. That was the year of a major tax reform act that owed its origin, if not its actual provisions, to a small group in the House of Representatives who were convinced that most U.S. philanthropic foundations were little more than tax dodges for millionaires, that the largest of them were controlled by self-appointed, self-perpetuating, elitist groups more interested in politics than in charity, and that their funds were dispersed as much to support questionable ideologies as to serve public interests.

As they had been in 1913 and 1928 and repeatedly thereafter, philanthropists and institutions supported by philanthropic donations were certain that the 1969 reform spelled doom for their beneficences and their hopes. It did indeed cause distress among givers and receivers alike. And it still does, to some extent. Yet a year after the act was passed, one of the nation's leading certified public accounting firms made this assessment of its impact: "The ardor of some donors toward charitable giving may have been cooled by premature lamentations by some that the 1969 act has emasculated the code provisions allowing the tax benefits previously available. Such is not the case. The act accomplished the closure of some 'loopholes' that generally were conceded to be such, but it also liberalized the rules in some areas back to reality. All things considered, charitable giving is still viable, and it will survive."[1]

It did survive, and had more than doubled again by 1978, when the total reached $39 billion, hampered in some respects by another reform act in 1976, which had elements of robbing Peter to pay Paul and about which the same CPA firm commented: "The wealthy have been affected substantially, and nearly all in this category will suffer greater gift and estate transfer costs. The new estate and gift provisions are complex and will need a plethora of clarifying regulations and rulings. The estate owner and his advisers face a real challenge to comprehend the impact of these revisions and react accordingly. Full understanding of the impact may take many years to accomplish.''[2] Some of the ambiguities in the act have been cleared up, and some remain.

Meanwhile, a committee of the Congress in 1978 considered and rejected a proposal that would have eliminated itemized income tax deductions entirely for an estimated six million taxpayers and was thus seen as a serious threat to philanthropic causes of all kinds. Later, a new and presumably more conservative Congress was expected to look with some favor on a bill that would protect against any further changes in the income tax code that would eliminate or inhibit tax encouragement of major philanthropy. Another provision of the bill would protect gifts to hospital operating funds and unrestricted gifts from being offset against expenses that would otherwise be reimbursed by government in publicly funded federal programs such as Medicare and Medicaid. Still another provision would amend the National Health Planning and Resources Development Act of 1974 to prohibit federal grants to health planning agencies in states promulgating legislation permitting use of such unrestricted gifts as an offset against state Medicaid payments.

"In this period of cost containment and in desperation to hold costs down, various state legislatures have proposed laws which would include charitable revenues as revenues subject to state control," warned James F. Clarke, former chairman of the governmental affairs committee of the National Association for Hospital Development, who played a major role in getting the Voluntary Hospital-Medical Center Philanthropic Support Bill drafted and introduced in the Congress in January 1979. "This sort of legislation, if adopted generally, would eventually put an end to philanthropic support for hospitals. It would serve no purpose other than to injure hospitals. By prohibiting grants in states that have adopted such a policy, Congress removes its support for such policies. The willingness of persons in the community to donate their money and time to voluntary not-for-profit hospitals results from and helps to perpetuate a sense of pride in the accomplishments of community hospitals that government regulation could never replace."[3]

Clarke wasn't just crying wolf. In defining "reasonable financial requirements" for the reimbursable cost base for hospitals, the Massachusetts Rate Setting Commission, a state agency, proposed that gift income be included as revenue applicable as reimbursement for the cost of service to Medicaid patients, a practice that would make government, not patients, the beneficiary of philanthropy. Hospital representatives vigorously opposed this subversion of the philanthropic purpose, and the commission withdrew the proposal for hospital rate submissions for 1978 but left the option open for the following year.

In a message to the commission aimed at forestalling renewal of the proposal, the New England Association for Hospital Development argued not only that it would obstruct the purposes of donors, interfere with the fiduciary responsibility of hospital trustees to decide how hospital funds should be used, and result in the ultimate demise of hospital philanthropy and its many benefits to society, but also that it might well be illegal. "As a governmental agency, the commission in its action to confiscate gift income relieves the government of the obligation to pay hospitals under the Medicaid program," the association pointed out. "Such action may constitute an unconstitutional taking of private property without just compensation." Besides, the association added, if all philanthropic initiative were to be extinguished, a consequence that could be expected to result from such action by government, "the basic needs of hospitals that are met presently through contributions will decrease, and these requirements will then be passed along through increased rate requests that will have to be met by the state."[4]

It isn't just hospitals that have felt threatened by reformers who want limits on the charitable tax deduction and restrictions on the use of charitable funds. In 1973, through the initiative of John D. Rockefeller III, Wilbur D. Mills, then chairman of the House Ways and Means Committee, and others, the Commission on

Private Philanthropy and Public Needs was organized with private and public support to examine the performance of nonprofit enterprise, or the third sector, as it has been called, to identify its position in the economy, set apart from both government and private business. The commission was headed by John H. Filer, chairman of the Aetna Life and Casualty Company, and its 31 members included "a diversity of views and a range of experiences encompassing the mainstream of American society,"[5] according to the commission staff. However, a coalition of public interest, social action, and volunteer groups that acted as advisers to the commission saw the members as "chosen overwhelmingly from among prominent businessmen, judges, religious leaders, university presidents, and foundation executives."[6] Inevitably under the circumstances, the commission's recommendations to the Congress, the findings and conclusions of its 91 separate research studies, and the 3,000-page report resulting from two years of investigation and deliberation have been subject to varying interpretations. Not surprisingly, the recommendations for the most part had to do with changes in the law that would amend the tax structure to encourage rather than further restrict tax incentives for giving to charitable causes by persons at all income levels. Based on extensive research studies by the commission staff and selected consultants reporting and estimating the effects of tax deductions on amounts donated to charitable causes, the recommendations among other things would:

- Permit all taxpayers who take the standard deduction to deduct charitable contributions also as a separate item, a recommendation that has already been introduced in the Congress.
- Permit families with incomes of less than $15,000 a year to deduct twice the amount of their charitable contributions and families with incomes from $15,000 to $20,000 to deduct 150 percent of contributions.
- Retain the appreciated property allowance in the charitable deductions, but eliminate any possibility of personal financial gain by giving.
- Retain the charitable bequest deduction.
- Require large tax-exempt organizations other than churches to make detailed annual reports on their finances and programs available.

- Require large grant-making organizations to hold public meetings annually to discuss their programs and contributions.
- Repeal the 4 percent audit tax on private foundations and replace it with fees based on audit costs.
- Establish a new category of independent foundations having the tax benefits of public charities but having a majority of governing board members unrelated to the foundation's benefactor or his family or business associates.
- Require all tax-exempt organizations to maintain arm's-length business relationships with profit-making organizations or activities in which any member of the organization's staff or board or any major contributor has a substantial financial interest.
- Establish a system of federal regulation of interstate charitable solicitations.

In addition to these and other recommendations for changes in federal law, the commission also proposed that "tax-exempt organizations recognize an obligation to be responsive to changing viewpoints and emerging needs and take steps such as broadening their boards and staffs to ensure responsiveness."[7] Finally, the commission recommended that corporations set as a minimum goal, to be reached no later than 1980, 2 percent of pre-tax net income for contributions to charitable purposes, and that a permanent national commission on the nonprofit sector should be established to conduct and stimulate ongoing research and generally to focus public attention on the significance of the voluntary sector in the national economy.

The advisory coalition of consumer organizations, or donee group, as it came to be called, came into existence when the commission was publicly criticized, at the midpoint of its studies, for focusing its attention on the concerns of givers to the virtual neglect of the needs of recipients, meaning both the recipients of services supported by philanthropic donations as well as institutions receiving the gifts and providing the services.

Responding to the criticism, the commission assembled the public-interest organizations that became the donee group and

asked them to review the studies and make their own comments
and recommendations. Noting that the commission had centered
its deliberations largely on technical tax considerations, the group
suggested that the perspective should be enlarged to comprehend
who benefits, and who should benefit, from private philanthropy.
In its report, which was published in 1977 as part of the six-volume
commission report, the donee group concluded that access to the
philanthropic process should be made more readily available to
many organizations now excluded from the system, that greater
accountability and changes in governance of voluntary institutions
are needed, that the donor community should be broadened by
giving everybody incentives to allocate money to charity, and that
"the present system of government regulation and control of
philanthropic organizations must be overhauled to eliminate im-
pediments to certain necessary activities and to provide exempt
organizations with competent, conscientious, and nonpartisan
oversight and supervision."[8]

The critical role for philanthropy in the future should be support of organizations monitoring, overseeing, or seeking changes
in government, industry, and other established institutions, the
group proposed. "We do not believe that philanthropy should
have as its primary purpose the support of private institutions performing essential services that are being delivered by business or
government," the report said. "Higher education, health care, the
arts, and other functions may be performed by public or private
institutions. In either case, it is done largely with public rather than
private funds. Since the amounts available from philanthropy for
support of service organizations will never be equal to the task
those organizations must undertake, philanthropy must consider
altering its objects of support to make optimum use of its limited
resources. It can do this by applying relatively small amounts of
money to social change, monitoring, and oversight functions
which can have long-lasting impact of greater significance. Philanthropy will have to actively seek objects of support rather than
remaining essentially passive while supporting established institutions."

Specific donee recommendations in pursuit of these goals had to
do for the most part with grant-making, rather than recipient, in-

stitutions and sought to broaden boards, require disclosures, limit tax exemptions, and avoid conflicts of interest. Other proposals were to add a substantial minimum tax to prevent higher-income taxpayers from avoiding taxation through use of deductions and provide more deductions and tax credits to encourage giving at lower-income levels.

Although it didn't seem likely that the donee group's recommendations would be considered seriously by a Congress thought to be more conservative than its predecessors, it wasn't by any means certain that the commission's recommendations would be either. Still, sponsors of the proposals to add a charitable deduction for standard deduction users and protect against state use of contributed funds had hopes that their bills, at least, would find some strong support. Whatever its strength, the support would owe something to extensive commission studies of the impact of taxation on giving. Thus a commission study by the Survey Research Center at the Institute for Social Research, University of Michigan, graphically demonstrated how giving as a percentage of income rises steeply starting with incomes in the $50,000 range, where the greater tax advantages begin to occur, and peaking at $250,000 to $500,000.

But it isn't true that big earners and big givers account for the largest share of all philanthropy, as they do, for example, in hospital capital gift campaigns. "Upper-income households give more absolutely and more even in relation to income," said the Michigan investigators, "but they are a small portion of all households. The result is that the bulk of aggregate giving comes from households with moderate incomes. More than half the total comes from households with incomes between $10,000 and $30,000, and they are nearly half of all households in the country."[9]

Hospital campaigns, on the other hand, commonly are based on a time-tested formula anticipating that 40 to 50 percent of the total should come from the top 10 gifts and another 35 to 40 percent from the next largest 100. Thus hospitals have an interest in holding onto the tax incentive for high incomes—and perhaps an untapped potential in adding incentives at the moderate and lower end of the scale. Most of the charitable giving of lower-income families now goes to their churches, the Michigan study found. "As income rises, people give more to the church, but they also expand the number of other charities they give to and presumably their motives for giving," the Michigan report said. An astonishing finding of the Michigan survey was that very few people knew their tax rate on the last dollar earned or the tax saving of giving another dollar to charity. "Mostly they only know whether they can get some advantage from itemizing," the researchers reported, adding that "of course, very high-income people are somewhat more likely to get expert help and a little more likely to know their tax rates."[10]

In a series of econometric studies conducted for the commission, which have been widely quoted and used to demonstrate the significant impact of tax incentives on giving, Harvard economics professor Martin S. Feldstein and several associates have shown that any increases in the price or net cost of giving will reduce the total of contributions received by charitable organizations by more than it increases the taxes collected by the Treasury Department. "The current deductibility of charitable gifts is a very efficient incentive," they concluded, "yielding more in additional gifts than the Treasury forgoes in potential additional revenues."[11] Another study for the commission demonstrated that tax incentives to encourage giving by low- and middle-income households would induce a substantial increase in the flow of funds to charitable institutions.[12] A third study concluded that over a wide range of estate size, charitable bequests are quite sensitive to the price reduction created by their deductibility.[13]

While the commission studies reported in detail the steady rise in giving to all charities over the years, the commission was obviously aware that the rise in dollars had barely kept up with the inflation, and in some years had fallen behind, and that over the past 20 years the public sector had begun to assume the initiative from private philanthropic institutions. "Decreasing levels of private giving, increasing costs of nonprofit activity, and broadening expectations for health, education, and welfare services as basic entitlements of citizenship have led to the government's becoming a principal provider of programs and revenues in many areas once dominated by private philanthropy," the commission report said, precisely describing the circumstance that had led to its creation. "Government's growing role in these areas poses fundamental questions about the autonomy and basic functioning of private nonprofit organizations and institutions."[14]

The commission may have come as close as anybody else has come, or could come, to answering the fundamental question of institutional autonomy and basic function of private nonprofit hospitals in a time of social upheaval: "Perhaps the most effective, and most possible, safeguard of autonomy is to have more than one purse to draw from," the report said. "The presence of a firm core of private support, however small, in a private organization that gets major public funding can be of crucial importance in determining whether the managers of the organization regard themselves, and behave, as independent operators or as civil servants."[15]

Keeping the critically important firm core of private support may not be easy at a time of decline in the propensity to give, as noted in one of the commission's research papers. One of the findings of a study by Ralph Nelson of Queens College, New York City, was a decline in the financial commitment to religious organizations, and particularly parochial schools, which he considered might be a result of the growth of public support of programs in education, health, welfare, and cultural activities perceived by potential contributors as substitutes for private support. "These and other factors may be shaping the attitudes of the cohorts of younger families who, while forming an increasing part of the economic base of giving, have developed giving habits different from, and usually less generous than, those of the cohorts of older families, who are a declining part of the economic base," Nelson said.[16]

In health care, it is the built-in limitations of public support that make retention of private support so important, in the opinion of another commission consultant, Robert J. Blendon, M.D., vice-president of the Robert Wood Johnson Foundation of Princeton, New Jersey. The public sector tends to move slowly and along traditional lines, and arrives only with difficulty at decisions to try new approaches, shrinking from the need to raise additional tax revenues, Blendon said. Inevitably, too, the public sector tends to shift health responsibilities from local to state and federal levels, thus diminishing the opportunities for local and individual initiatives. Moreover, public bodies are restrained from responding to the legitimate wishes of particular religious, ethnic, and other special interests to have health services designed and provided for their own special needs.

"Because of these very real limitations that are inevitably a part of the public sector process, it will be in the public interest to encourage the continued tax exemption of philanthropic gifts in the health field," Blendon concluded. "A major strength of our nation is the active participation of multiple groups in our public affairs. It seems particularly important to preserve and foster pluralistic sources of support in the health area. It is not enough for Americans to recognize the need for long-term change and evolution in our system for developing medical science and applying it to the health concerns of our citizens. We must have an institutional climate that can make such changes possible. It is around this issue that the case for private philanthropy in health rests. Without a viable philanthropic sector in health, all future innovations, new ideas, and scientific theories would have but one possible source of support—the relatively centralized public sector, which is not designed for such a role."[17]

The way things have turned out, whether or not we shall have a viable philanthropic sector in health for the future may be as much a political as a philosophic question. It is a time of political volatility, and uncertainty is the norm. But for the time being, at least, philanthropy marches on. Its supporters are busier than ever in Washington and the state capitals, seeking to fend off further inroads on charitable deductions and restrictions on use of charitable donations. And when they get home, they are busier than ever identifying and cultivating givers and obtaining gifts. Surprisingly, in view of all the pressures their efforts have never been more productive for health care, whose 15 percent of 1978's $39 million bounty was second only to religious causes, which have stirred the most people to give the most money ever since the Good Samaritan paid the wounded traveler's bill at the inn. As one might expect, hospitals get the largest share of the health care charitable dollar.

It is a disquieting fact, however, that private giving for some years has been a diminishing fraction of the total amount spent building and operating hospitals. The reason is not so much that interest among givers has lagged as that money from other sources, notably government and insurance, has risen dramatically. In one recent study, philanthropy was reported as contributing less than 9 percent of all money spent for hospital construction; government grants were 23 percent, debt financing was 57 percent, and the rest came from earned reserves.[18]

Thus philanthropy marches on still, but there can be no denying that the sound of the trumpets is muted. "It isn't so much that anything drastic has happened yet," said a fund raiser who manages capital gift campaigns for hospitals, principally in the Eastern states where the philanthropic tradition has its firmest roots and where state rate review threatening retention and use of philanthropic funds is making the most waves. "Some of the proposed rules would amount to confiscation of hospital funds," the fund raiser said, "and I can't believe the legislatures will go along with these proposals. But some hospital boards are intimidated. They feel that almost anything could happen, and that keeps them from going ahead with plans to modernize, or replace old buildings, or invest in new equipment, much less to expand. It's rarely a question of adding beds any more. It's a matter of maintaining quality. A lot of hospitals aren't doing it."

Such fears are not unreasonable. Some members of the Congress are known to be opposed to any kind of philanthropic support of health and education, not for the ideological reasons that surfaced during the 1969 debate about tax reform but because of the real loss of tax revenues represented in the charitable income tax deduction. And some lawmakers and influential bureaucrats consider that philanthropic gifts to hospitals are especially objectionable. Contributions supporting an added facility or service, they believe, are in effect private decisions that commit expenditures of public funds under existing and future entitlements. Such expenditures presumably would be allowed only to the extent that added services or facilities are approved by the appropriate certificate-of-need or planning authority, it is acknowledged, but these processes are not always effective. In any case, there would always be added costs representing private disposition of public resources.

The countervailing argument is simply that the whole purpose of philanthropy, like the purpose of tax exemption for eleemosynary institutions, is to establish and encourage private means for the achievement of socially desirable goals. Thus the lost tax revenues and any other expenses are returned, with generous dividends, through support of institutions performing functions that would have to be provided and paid for by government if the institutions did not exist and the voluntary private support were not forth-coming. The scope of this argument has been narrowed somewhat by the advent of Medicare and Medicaid, but it is by no means vitiated, since there are many services required by eligible program beneficiaries that are not provided under Medicare and Medicaid, and many costs to providing institutions that are not fully paid in the programs.

Nobody knows which arguments may prevail or just what restraints may be legislated in the future. Forecasting what the Congress and the states may do is an imprecise art even for the most seasoned of political observers, and a perilous ground for decision-making even for the most provident of hospital boards. Meanwhile, however, most hospital boards, like the governing bodies of churches, universities, academies, museums, and other enterprises depending in some part on philanthropic funds, are moving ahead with their fund-raising activities, however nervously. Whatever happens, they are convinced that charitable donations will never be completely outlawed, and as long as they can per-suade people to give, it is better to have than to have not. In 1979, they got $6 billion for medical institutions.

How? The methods hospitals use to get money are described in detail in the remaining chapters of this book, but a few observa-tions about the state of the art may be appropriate here. The asking business, like most occupations in a complex society, has its own special body of knowledge and rules of practice, but the root responsibility for organizing and directing the effort resides with hospital trustees. However much of this burden they may delegate to others, it is trustees who have to do most of the asking. The essence of the art of raising money is matching askers to givers, so that on every occasion where it is at all possible the former will be the one person best suited to evoke the right response from the latter. And since the greater share of the money lies in the territory, or social stratum, from which the greater number of hospital trustees are recruited, more often than not the one person best suited to evoke the right response is going to be a trustee.

Whoever it is, the trustee or physician or volunteer who objects that "I simply can't ask for money!" or "I'm not any good at this!" should be taken seriously but not relieved of the responsibility. However shy a person may be about making the presentation and asking for money, he or she may still play a central role in arranging meetings, making introductions, and accompanying someone else who may actually ask for the money during a call. If the trustee is genuinely interested in the hospital and its mission, in time this enthusiasm for the cause will usually outrun any shyness and the trustee may become an effective money raiser. If what his protest actually means is that the trustee really isn't interested enough to undertake an assignment that doesn't appeal to him particularly, then he certainly should be excused from the fund-raising task, if not from the board, because belief in the institutional mission is essential to voluntary service. There is no substitute for dedication as an effective fund-raising instrument.

In the past, the greater part of the money that dedicated fund raisers have moved into hospitals has gone to build buildings, and because buildings are visible and long lasting, the practice of memorializing donors and their families in stone and steel has made the name on the building or wing or floor or room as familiar to the hospital culture as meal trays and nurses' uniforms. Development officers have made the memorial approach an art form, and that is one reason they are so apprehensive about the outlook for hospital philanthropy as they consider the public pronouncements about too many hospitals and too many beds, the public laws and regulations with curbs on building, and the public proposals for limits on capital expansion of any kind. But even if all the curbs were to be effected, as some of them have been, there are still going to be new hospital buildings to replace those that are wearing out. Even if there were to be no new buildings or equip-

CHAPTER 3

Asking and Giving: In the Beginning

Although it is likely that the cavemen shared such comforts as they enjoyed on occasion, and anthropologists have recorded aboriginal behavior exhibiting charity and love among primitive tribes, the earliest evidence of philanthropy as an organized force in society goes back to the pharoahs of ancient Egypt, who were known to have established perpetuities to ensure the support of religious rites and practices. That was 3,000 years ago, give or take. A few centuries later Plato, a rich man who valued wisdom and justice ahead of property, founded his Academy for the pursuit of philosophic and scientific knowledge. When he died in 347 B.C., Plato bequeathed lands to his nephew Speusippus for continued support of the Academy, which endured until the emperor Justinian, who considered such academies threatening, closed them and appropriated their emoluments, possibly setting a precedent for political thought and conduct that are not unknown in our own time. But the rulers of Greece and Rome were not without charity; they often gave lands to the poor, constructed public gardens for the enrichment of life, and sponsored public feasts and entertainments.

The word *philanthropy,* which simply means "love of mankind," did not come into common use until the 17th or 18th century. But *charity,* or the Greek *agape,* is used interchangeably with *love* in the New Testament. Early Roman law had rules of charity defining the duties owed to guests and neighbors and rules for providing shelter for strangers. St. Augustine held charity to be the "root of all virtue" that linked man to God. But the most celebrated of all the concepts elevating charity, or love, above all other human values has to be the eloquent lyric of St. Paul's epistle to the Corinthians:

Though I speak with the tongues of men and of angels, and have not charity, I am become as sounding brass, or a tinkling cymbal.

And though I have the gift of prophecy, and understand all mysteries, and all knowledge, and though I have all faith, so that I could remove mountains, and have not charity, I am nothing.

And though I bestow all my goods to feed the poor, and though I give my body to be burned, and have not charity, it profiteth me nothing.

Charity suffereth long, and is kind; charity envieth not; charity vaunteth not itself; is not puffed up,

Doth not behave itself unseemly, seeketh not her own, is not easily provoked, thinketh no evil;

Rejoiceth not in iniquity, but rejoiceth in the truth;

Beareth all things, believeth all things, hopeth all things, endureth all things.

Charity never faileth: but whether there be prophecies, they shall fail; whether there be tongues, they shall cease; whether there be knowledge, it shall vanish away.

For we know in part, and we prophesy in part.

But when that which is perfect is come, then that which is in part shall be done away.

When I was a child, I spake as a child, I understood as a child, I thought as a child; but when I became a man, I put away childish things.

For now we see through a glass, darkly; but then face to face, now I know in part; but then shall I know even as also I am known.

And now abideth faith, hope, charity, these three; but the greatest of these is charity.

In a later message to the Corinthians, Paul was more explicit about the duties and rewards of charity when he said: "Every man according as he purposeth in his heart, so let him give; not grudgingly, or of necessity: for God loveth a cheerful giver. He hath dispersed abroad, he hath given to the poor: his righteousness remaineth forever."

The teachings of Christ and his followers echoed the earlier exhortations of the Jewish prophets, as of Isaiah, who said: "Is it not to deal thy bread to the hungry, and that thou bring the poor to thy house? When thou seest the naked that thou cover him? Then shall thy light break forth as the morning, and thine health shall spring forth speedily, and thy righteousness shall go before thee; the glory of the Lord shall be thy reward."

The Mosaic law specifically enjoined man always to show consideration for his less fortunate brothers. A 12th-century leader of Jewish thought, the great physician and philosopher Maimonides, defined the degrees of grace to be gained through the varying circumstances and intentions of giving:

1. Giving less than is needed, without kindness.
2. Giving less than is needed, but with good grace.
3. Giving after a request is made.
4. Giving where donor and recipient know each other but the gift is made before it is requested.
5. Giving so that the recipient knows the donor.
6. Giving so that the donor knows the recipient.
7. Giving charity to the poor so that neither the donor nor the recipient knows the other.
8. Helping the needy to be independent by providing opportunity for work or advancing loans.

It is doubtful that these niceties of intention and recognition could be applied to much of the charitable giving of modern society, where the donor must always be known to someone and the recipient of the gift is usually an intermediary institution or organization, and not the ultimate beneficiary. But the meaning of Maimonides is nonetheless clear: the act of giving is most elevated when the intention is most selfless.

But there is a benign kind of selfishness, or self-involvement, that has been at the core of religiously motivated philanthropy over all the years and was described by a 2nd-century Christian teacher, St. Clement of Alexandria: " Charity, as man's love for man, should be based not on the desirability of its object but on the transformation of its subject through the power of divine agape," wrote St. Clement. In a "discourse concerning the salvation of rich men, a tract on the use of wealth," St. Clement took a clear-eyed view of possessions, which he said should be regarded as instruments to be used either for good or evil purposes. "The word does not command us to renounce property but to manage property," he wrote, urging that alms should be dispensed with discernment to the deserving needy.

Throughout the early years of the Christian era, and in fact persisting beyond the Reformation and probably still observable in some giving for religious causes, some ecclesiastics have turned St. Clement's concept of "transformation through the power of divine agape" inside out to serve their own fund-raising purposes. Thus rich landowners in the Middle Ages were persuaded that generous gifts to help build churches, monasteries, and hospices would surely earn them passports to heaven; for a price, the sinner could buy forgiveness for his sins, of whatever magnitude. The sale of indulgences became widespread and was often abused by priests who lived like princes while the needs of the poor were neglected. It was denounced by Martin Luther and diminished following the Reformation, but has probably never disappeared altogether.

The fact that the sale of indulgences was abused by venal churchmen, however, does not denigrate the charities of those givers who were convinced that their good works would earn them God's favor or of those who sincerely believed that their wealth was a gift of God that should be returned to serve His purposes—a belief that, according to members of his family and many others, was the chief reason for the legendary philanthropies of John D. Rockefeller. In *The Vision of Piers Plowman,* the epic tale of a search for truth in 14th-century England, the wealthy are advised to seek forgiveness by using their fortunes to "repair hospitals, help sick people, mend bad roads, build up bridges, find food for prisoners and poor people, put scholars to school or to some other craft, help religious orders, and ameliorate rents or taxes.''

The Elizabethan poor laws initiated the as yet uncompleted process of making the care and well-being of the less fortunate the concern of the state instead of only the church. The first poor law levied a rate on all householders to provide for the poor and was said to be the first legal and secular obligation in addition to the recognized moral and religious duties to give alms. Elizabeth's law was followed by others in the 17th-century, and later, but as always happens, the poor outran the state and multiplied faster than the laws and the charities could. Nevertheless, the concept that charity was ''lending to the Lord, who in good time will return the gift with increase,'' as Calvinist reformers had it, persisted, and charities increased along with trade and prosperity.

At the same time, there were many who gave alms as an alternative to paying increased tribute to the crown, a choice not unlike the one faced by today's high-tax-bracket philanthropists. Then as now, too, feelings about the poor were mixed. Some saw them as neglected or forgotten children of God, deserving whatever help the state and the charitably inclined could give them, while others considered alms as thrown away on the idle, the wicked, and the worthless. ''The lower classes must be kept poor, or they will never be industrious'' was a common attitude in 18th- and 19th-century England and on the continent, and it wasn't unknown in America. ''People ought to be healthy. If they ain't healthy they can't work, and if they don't work they ain't healthy, and if they can't work there ain't no profit in them,'' said James Buchanan Duke, founder of the Duke Endowment, a bountiful supporter of health institutions and causes since the 1920s.[1]

Elizabeth I and her Tudor predecessors had been jealous, if not fearful, of the church's wealthy holdings and had encouraged the formation of private charitable corporations by law and by royal charter. The endowments of these forerunners of today's foundations were used to establish and support universities and hospitals, some of which are still in existence. The same period saw the early origins of the private charitable trust, some formed for meritorious causes and some simply to perpetuate the crotchets of the rich. In European countries dominated by the Catholic

Church, kings and princes were even more fearful of the wealth and power of the church and generally sought to keep closer controls on all distributions of private capital—again, a practice traces of which are still discernible.

When he wasn't busy arranging divorces, Henry VIII had time to become interested in and to endow St. Bartholomew's Hospital of London, which was then already 400 years old. But charitable hospitals were nothing new even when St. Bart's was founded in 1123. The Hotel Dieu at Lyons, in France, began in A.D. 542. The early Christians of Rome had established hospitals for lepers, cripples, the blind, and the sick poor, and European explorers in the Middle Ages helped the religious brotherhoods and sisterhoods create asylums in connection with their monasteries and convents. The Hospital of Jesus of Nazareth in Mexico City was founded by Cortez in 1524. The oldest hospital in North America is the Hotel Dieu of Quebec, established in 1639. The Hotel Dieu of Montreal started five years later.

In the United States, where there has never been a single all-powerful government or church establishment, philanthropy has flourished nevertheless as an expression of the charitable impulse of free men and women, either as individuals or collectively in voluntary associations. "Wherever at the head of some new undertaking you see the government in France or a man of rank in England, in the United States you will be sure to find an association," Alexis de Tocqueville wrote in 1845. "The Americans make associations to give entertainments, to found seminaries, to build inns, to construct churches, to diffuse books, to send missionaries to the Antipodes; in this manner they found hospitals, prisons and schools."[2]

As this suggests, voluntary associations in the United States are not opposed to but often linked to religion. Many of the associations and benevolent societies are organized for and devoted to church or other religious purposes. The relationship is not accidental. The traditions of hard work, thrift, and devotion to family and community laid down by the early settlers were closely tied to their religious beliefs. "The acquisition of riches is to them only a help toward higher spiritual and moral ends,"[3] said another 19th-century visitor to America, Philip Schaff a Swiss theologian, and a contemporary observer has explained further. "The emphasis on voluntarism in both areas, religious and secular, has clearly been mutually reinforcing," said Seymour Martin Lipset of Stanford University. "Men were expected to be righteous, hardworking, and ambitious. Righteousness was to be rewarded both in the present and the hereafter, and the successful had an obligation to engage in good works and to share the bounty they had attained."[4]

Hard work and good works were virtues shared by the founders of the first hospital in the American colonies. Like hundreds of other hospitals that were to follow in the United States, the Pennsylvania Hospital of Philadelphia was created in 1751 by the combined talents of a dedicated physician and an interested and influential man of affairs. The physician was Thomas Bond, a Maryland Quaker who was educated in London and Paris and returned to America to become Port Inspector for Contagious Diseases at Philadelphia. The man of affairs was Benjamin Franklin, who described the origins of the hospital, including the fund-raising tactic, in his celebrated *Autobiography:* "In 1751 Dr. Thomas Bond, a particular friend of mine, conceived the idea of establishing a hospital in Philadelphia (a very beneficent design, which has been ascribed to me but was originally and truly his) for the reception and cure of poor sick persons, whether inhabitants of the province or strangers. He was zealous and active in endeavoring to procure subscriptions for it; but the proposal being a novelty in America, and at first not well understood, he met with but little success. At length he came to me with the compliment that he found there was no such thing as carrying a public-spirited project through without my being concerned in it. 'For' he said, 'I am often asked by those to whom I propose subscribing, "Have you consulted Franklin on this business? And what does he think of it?" And when I tell them I have not (supposing it rather out of your line), they do not subscribe but say they will consider it.' I inquired into the nature and utility of the scheme, and receiving a very satisfactory explanation, I not only subscribed to it myself but engaged heartily in the design of procuring subscriptions from others. Previously, however, to the solicitation, I endeavored to prepare the minds of the people by writing on the subject in the newspapers, which was my usual custom in such cases, but which he had omitted.

"The subscriptions afterwards were more free and generous; but beginning to flag, I saw they would be insufficient without some assistance from the Assembly, and, therefore, proposed to petition for it; which was done. The country members did not at first relish the project; they objected that it could only be serviceable to the city, and, therefore, the citizens alone should be at the expense of it; and they doubted whether the citizens themselves generally approved of it. My allegations to the contrary, that it met with such approbation as to leave no doubt of our being able to raise two thousand pounds by voluntary donations, they considered as a most extravagant supposition and utterly impossible. On this I formed my plan and asked leave to bring in a bill for incorporating the contributors . . . which leave was obtained chiefly on the condition that the House could throw the bill out if they did not like it. I drew it so as to make the important clause a conditional one, viz.: 'And be it enacted by the authority aforesaid that when the said contributors shall have met and chosen their managers and treasurer and shall have raised by their contributions a capital stock of two thousand pounds value, the yearly interest of which is to be applied to the accommodation of the sick poor in the said hospital, and free of charge for diet, attendance, advice, and medicines, and shall make the same appear to the satisfaction of the speaker of the Assembly; that then it shall and may be lawful for the said speaker, and he is hereby required to sign an order on the provincial treasurer for the payment of two thousand pounds in two yearly payments, to the treasurer of the said hospital, to be applied to the founding, building, and finishing of the same.'

"This condition carried the bill through; for the members who had opposed the grant, and now conceived they might have the credit of being charitable without the expense, agreed to its passage; and then in soliciting subscriptions among people, we urged the conditional promise of the law as an additional motive to give, since every man's donation would be doubled; thus the cause worked both ways. The subscriptions accordingly soon exceeded the requisite sum, and we claimed and received the public gift, which enabled us to carry the design into execution. A convenient and handsome building was soon erected, the institution has by constant experience been found useful, and I do not remember any of my political maneuvers, the success of which at the time gave me more pleasure; or wherein, after thinking of it, I more easily excused myself for having made use of some cunning."[5]

In another sequence that has been repeated over and over in the history of many if not most hospitals, the Pennsylvania Hospital within three years of opening its doors found itself in need of more cash, and the managers asked Franklin to "prepare a full account of the affairs of the Hospital to be laid before the Assembly." In *Some Account of the Pennsylvania Hospital,* the resulting 40-page tract of which 1,500 copies were printed and distributed in the community, he argued that the institution was not only a deserving charity but a prudent investment, a means by which "the distress of the distempered poor" could be relieved so that they might be "restored to Health and Comfort and become useful to themselves, their Families and the Publick, for many years after." There had been reason to expect a considerable subscription toward the support of such a hospital, Franklin wrote, "but the Expense of erecting a Building sufficiently large and commodious for the Purpose, it was thought would be too heavy, unless the Subscription could be made general throughout the Province." On its final page the tract included a subscription form. Within a few months the hospital had added 186 new subscribers who donated another £2,000.[6]

Franklin was a frequent contributor to the hospital and served on its board of managers until he left the country, and he made a bequest to the hospital in his will. But for him, doing good was a duty of citizenship, not of piety. "The gospel of industry, frugality, and sobriety was worldly wisdom rather than spiritual discipline," Robert H. Bremner, professor of history at Ohio State University, wrote in a paper on the history of philanthropy, relating also that Franklin once acknowledged that the guiding influence in his philanthropies had been Cotton Mather's *Essays To Do Good.*[7] Published in 1710, this best known of Mather's voluminous writings urged people to a perpetual endeavor to do good in the world, not only as an obligation owed to God but as a matter of sound social policy. A generous philanthropist himself and a founder of Yale University, Mather was convinced that "those who devote themselves to good devices usually find a

wonderful increase of their opportunities,'' but he also considered
that the wealthy had an obligation to give wisely. ''Let us try to do
good with as much application of mind as wicked men employ in
doing evil,'' he said, and there can be little doubt that if this advice
had been followed more scrupulously in our own time, ''doing
good'' could never have come to be a term of derision, as it often
has been.

In addition to his own charities and his prodigious output of
books, pamphlets, and sermons, Cotton Mather was known in
Boston as a tireless promoter of benevolent societies for a variety
of civic and religious purposes. His example caught on and
resulted in the proliferation of associations remarked a century
later by deTocqueville. ''As early as 1820 the larger cities had an
embarrassment of benevolent organizations,'' wrote Bremner, and
indeed, as it turns out, ours was not the first generation to look on
''doing good'' as a mark of opprobrium. ''Emerson warned the
'foolish philanthropist' not to come to his door begging for 'your
miscellaneous popular charities; the educational colleges of fools;
the building of meeting houses to the vain end to which many now
stand; alms to sots, and the thousand-fold Relief Societies.' For
the rest of the century, and even to our own day, one of the major
problems of charity reformers would be to discover ways to coordinate the activities and fund drives of these competing
agencies.''[8]

Throughout much of the 19th century, the chief goal of philanthropy for hospitals remained the provision of shelter and medical
care for the sick poor, prompted in part by the humanitarian
desire to relieve suffering and in part by the prudent wish to make
them productive members of society and relieve the burden on
poorhouses and poor farms supported by local authorities.
Medical colleges had been founded at Philadelphia, Harvard, and
King's College (later Columbia University) in New York City in
the late 1700s, and medical students learned and practiced their
skills in the wards of the great charitable hospitals then, as they do
now. But it was more than a century later before medical
education was to become a major objective of philanthropy in the
United States.

Meanwhile, the function of hospitals as something more than a refuge for the sick poor began to broaden with the advancement of medical science, and chiefly the discovery of anesthesia in 1848, Lister's work in antisepsis in 1865, and Roentgen's discovery of X rays in 1895. These monumental achievements, among others, made surgery a preferred modality of treatment for a multitude of diseases and conditions, instead of a final recourse for the desperate, and initiated the linking of businessmen who were making fortunes in growing new industries and surgeons who needed facilities for the exercise of their skills and the welfare of their patients. As Bond and Franklin had done a century earlier, dedicated physicians and wealthy benefactors were seeking and finding each other all over the country, and it was this combination, or some variation of it, that fueled the early growth and development of the voluntary hospital system in the United States and that has remained a distinctive and important characteristic of the system ever since.

CHAPTER 4

The Asking Business

Fund raising is big business. In 1978, $39 billion was contributed to voluntary institutions and organizations in the United States. The proportion of that amount that resulted from some systematic effort on the part of the recipients is not known, but it is certain that not very much of it could have slipped unprompted and unaided from the hands of the donors into the coffers of the causes. Not many give without being asked, and asking is a billion dollar industry today.

Viewed as an industry, the asking business can be divided into three major sectors: the professional fund-raising consultants, specialists, and firms that advise and assist organizations and institutions in their fund-raising activities; the full-time fund-raising and development staff members on the organizational payrolls; and the vast army of executives, board and auxiliary members, and volunteers for whom raising money is either a part-time duty, as for college presidents and priests, or a civic or religious obligation, as for trustees and auxiliary members.

Viewed another way, the asking industry can be seen as consisting of the annual request for sustaining funds, largely by mailings to extensively culled and cultivated lists; the intensive, short-term drive for capital funds; and the continuing, long-term development task of identifying, interesting, and influencing major donors. All three types of fund raising—annual, intensive, and long-term—involve all three types of fund raiser: professional adviser, full-time staff, and part-time executive and volunteer.

The annual campaign for gifts is a commonplace activity among colleges and hospitals. Often it is seasonal, as when colleges make their appeal to alumni at commencement and reunion times or hospitals canvass their constituencies near the end of the year, when the appeal for support can be accompanied by a reminder that the deadline for current tax deductions is at hand. In any case, the business of soliciting annual gifts for institutions is not a simple matter of dusting off last year's letter and last year's list and repeating the performance. If it is to be a significant source of institutional support—and for some hospitals it is a million dollar source, year after year—it requires a correspondingly significant effort in planning and preparing the appeal, coordinating the campaign with other fund-raising activities, and evaluating the results.

These are measured in dollars, to be sure, but there are other values to be assessed as well: the number of new donors, the number of former donors who failed to contribute, the number who increased their contributions, the size of gifts. All these and other details of campaign results are clues to the community's interest in and feeling for the institution. Increasing community interest and improving community attitude, along with financial support, are considered by most hospital and college executives to be important objectives of the annual gift campaign effort.

For some institutions, the annual campaign is an all-out push involving trustees, physicians, auxiliary members, and other volunteers calling on selected prospects, as is commonly done in capital fund drives. In most cases, however, this use of institutional resources and volunteers is focused on the solicitation of major gifts for specific objectives, and the annual campaign is conducted by mail.

Recently, some institutions have experimented with concentrated telephone appeals to selected prospects. For the past several years, for example, Ohio State University has conducted an intensive two-week telephone campaign using volunteers in 30 communities across the state to call OSU alumni and ask for gifts.

Other universities have used volunteer faculty members and students, or paid callers, in similar efforts. The method is perhaps not as applicable to hospitals, whose constituencies don't have the same kind of relationship to the institution that alumni are felt to have, but some hospital development officers consider that former patients and donors may be considered hospital "alumni" and some have used telephone solicitation of selected donors with reportedly satisfactory results.

When the annual campaign consists wholly of appeals by mail, however, it isn't much simpler. Building lists, keeping them current, adding new names, testing various kinds of appeals, achieving an appropriate balance of persuasive message and institutional need, and measuring results are tasks that require expert technical knowledge and creative skill. When these and other fund-raising assignments are relegated to someone in the organization without special training and knowledge, or someone with other duties as well, or, as is often the case, to a member of the auxiliary who is thought to have a flair for the colorful phrase, the results are likely to be disappointing. Under these circumstances, the board and the administration may readily decide that "There is no real opportunity for philanthropy as a source of support for hospitals any more, with taxes what they are today and the government interfering with everything." When that attitude prevails, for that institution it becomes a self-fulfilling prophecy.

When, on the other hand, fund raising is seen as a serious business and as much a part of institutional financial management as accounting for receivables and analyzing reimbursement formulas, the annual gift campaign is not something that can be tossed off to subordinates to handle when they aren't busy with something else. Rather, it is a first-line responsibility commanding attention from the board of trustees, where objectives are established and policies formulated, to the fund-raising staff, where the dimensions and details of the task are comprehended. The method may be the all-out effort, the telephone campaign, or only the mail appeal, but the planning, organization of resources, execution, and evaluation are as carefully conducted, by people who know what they're doing, as a major procedure in the operating room. And from the standpoint of institutional governance and management, one activity is as important as the other. Where this is the case, moreover, the annual campaign is not regarded as something apart from, and perhaps even competitive with, the intensive capital fund drive or the long-term development program. Instead, all three activities are seen as components of an ongoing, coordinated financial development plan.

The concept that the annual campaign is for nickels and dimes and is something major donors and prospects should be shielded from gives way to a structured approach that makes the annual appeal a preparation for, or supplement to, the major capital gift. "The essense of the annual fund is continuity," said a bulletin published by Gonser, Gerber, Tinker, and Stuhr, development consultants to educational and charitable organizations. "It should never be stopped. The goal should be wide participation as a means of getting donors acquainted with and involved in the institution's program. There should be specific goals and specific projects in the annual fund. The habit of annual giving is strong, and it should not be automatically assumed that gifts to an annual fund are smaller than gifts to a capital campaign. It all depends on the program and the motivation of the donor."[1]

Understanding the hospital's development program and the motivation of the donor is the key to success in any fund-raising endeavor, whatever the goal or the method may be, and the key to understanding is adequate research. In mail campaigns, the research is aimed at building and maintaining lists. It is likely that every hospital keeps a list of former patients who have made some contribution or have shown some interest in the institution, and most hospitals have a system for adding to the list by reviewing admissions and determining which families are judged to be prospective donors, using such clues as the residential address, the type of accommodation chosen, the employment information on the admissions form, and perhaps the method of payment. This core of people with known relationship to the hospital, along with trustees, physicians, auxiliary members, and selected employees, all of whom may appropriately be considered as prospects for annual gifts, is sure to add up to several hundred names even in the smallest communities. It may readily be several thousand in more populous areas, where lists may also include businesses whose employees use the hospital, residents of the service area other than former patients, and any who are known to be contributors to other charitable enterprises.

These are just beginnings. In cities, lists can be purchased or rented from publishers, merchants, utilities, and other sources, including list houses that are in the business of merchandising names. For relatively small amounts such lists can be tested to determine whether their use for the hospital's purpose would be productive. But the tests need to be conducted, and the lists supervised by a staff member or consultant who knows the techniques of list management and use. At today's postage rates, unproductive use of the mail is an expensive way to learn the business.

Raising money by mail isn't any longer a matter of sending a single, all-purpose letter to everybody on the list and then counting the checks as they come in. The wording of the appeal is known to have an impact on the result, for example, and direct mail experts have demonstrated that even the arrangement of paragraphs on the page can make a difference. In extensive campaigns, variations in the form of the appeal can be tested before whole lists are canvassed, and in such carefully planned and conducted efforts lists can be divided according to what is known about the prospects. In some cases, the extra expense of personally addressed letters may be fully justified. Or it may be that list research will suggest that some recipients would be more responsive to an appeal based on the hospital's emergency services, or research programs, or the needs of the pediatrics department. Again, sophisticated management is required for effective and economical fund raising as much as it is for engineering or personnel or any other phase of operations.

Increasingly, mail campaigns are conducted on a year-round basis instead of in a concentrated period at one time of year. At the Lenox Hill Hospital in New York City, for example, the program includes anniversary mailings with an appeal sent to the donor every year on the anniversary of his first gift, new patient mailings that are sent three months following the patients' discharges, emergency room mailings once a year to prospects who have used the hospital's emergency services, and year-end mailings to all those who have not responded to other appeals during the year. The year-end mailing is also used to test new audiences. Once lists have been established on computers, as sizable mail lists commonly are today—either in-house for large institutions or by computer service agencies for others, all these and other specialized mailing schedules and forms of appeal are easily managed.

"At Lenox Hill in the course of the last four years we have done much experimenting with the form of our appeals," said Jack Rimalover, assistant vice-president for resources development and public affairs, who has held similar positions at Columbia University and in business. "We have gone from multi-stuffer envelopes to single-sheet self-mailers to gimmicky, rip-off opener mailers, and this year to a unique questionnaire approach to our audiences. The results over the years indicate an increasing response to all our appeals, a higher dollar average per response, and an increasing percentage of return to each category of mailing."[2]

For his fellow members of the National Association for Hospital Development, Rimalover summed up what he considers to be the most practical way of making sure direct mail programs work as a "three-T" approach: testing, timing, and tabulating. On testing, he said, "You do not need tremendous samples to determine how your mailing will do. If you have the time to run a preliminary mailing, a small representative sample will show within a percent or two how your final mailing will turn out." Also, he added, "Test your list. The art of choosing lists is sophisticated. Consider getting help from professionals, including list brokers. Above all, do not be afraid to be innovative. Try to test lists that you think might work for your hospital."

Timing should also be tested, Rimalover advised, "At Lenox Hill we spread our mailings over most of the year. This reduces cost, reduces the year-end work load, and, most important, it spreads income over the year. But there is no easy answer to the best time to mail. The only way to find out what is best for your institution is to test your timing. If you are afraid of jeopardizing a successful mailing, test a piece of it at another time of the year. Only you can find out for yourself."

As for the third T, tabulating, Rimalover said, "All your efforts will be worthless if you do not keep records, analyze your results, and compile statistics. Which of your audiences have been most successful? You want to determine the percent return from one category to another. You may want to analyze average dollar and percent of returns from one time of year to another. Another important tabulation would enable you to check the performance of lists from year to year. For example, we have found that there is a considerable return from ex-patients if we keep after them for one or two years, but if they have not made a contribution by the time three years have passed, it is not worth going after them again. This year, we dropped 4,000 or 5,000 people from our list because of their very low rate of return." Finally, Rimalover concluded, "If there is any one most important rule in marketing, it is this: Ask for the order. Whether in person or by mail, state what you are after and give the recipient a chance to respond."

Another successful direct mail approach was described by Carryl R. Ziettlow, director of resource development, Iowa Methodist Medical Center, Des Moines, where a "Partners in Healing" appeal enrolls contributors as benefactors, colleagues, companions, or friends, according to the size of their gifts. Like Rimalover, Ziettlow believes in trying out different appeals, in using different tactics for different audiences and times of year, and in analyzing results. The mail approach to former patients consists of three letters, he explained. "We are experimenting now with two different types of letter for the first mailing," he said. "These are mailed within a month or two after the patient has been discharged. If there is no response after the first letter, the second letter is sent after a month or two. If there is no response at that time, we follow up with a deferred-giving letter, which gives them an opportunity to request information about our deferred gifts program."[3]

Ziettlow also gives former donors special treatment. "One of the expensive things in direct-mail fund raising is not following up on individuals once they have given," he said. "There are many who respond only when they are asked, and they must be asked repeatedly. For that reason, once or twice a year we mail a letter specifically designed to reactivate the past donor."

Iowa Methodist also makes special mailings to rural families throughout the state, and special holiday appeals at Christmas, Valentine's Day, and Mother's Day. Recognition is important for givers in all categories, Ziettlow believes, and once a year "we compile the names of all who have given to us on the various donor levels and publish them in a quality piece which we call our *Donor Appreciation Journal.* This is mailed to donors so they may look to see who their friends are who have given. We also make it available here at the medical center in the hope that it will encourage others to consider contributing, or moving to a different level."

The "Partners in Healing" idea has been used elsewhere, more successfully in some places than in others, a circumstance suggesting that its effectiveness is determined not so much by the particular device as by the way it is applied. Variations on this type of recognition have been used frequently, with good results, to encourage substantial donations on an annual basis by offering membership in exclusive clubs or societies to donors of $1,000 or more. At one university society membership is $10,000 a year, and there are 200 members.

John F. Donovan, director of development and public relations at the Salem (Massachusetts) Hospital, explained that the minimum gift society concept was initiated at an Ivy League university many years ago and has many different forms, but the premise is simple: "Each year, board members personally solicit three contributors for large total gifts payable over several tax years as annual contributions. Almost every board member should be able to participate in three solicitations a year. The major impetus is to create a special group separate from the board and other leadership groups. Universities from Harvard to Southern California have used this mechanism successfully to attract highly selected donors for predictable and substantial gifts. Although the value of the minimum gift society is the generation of annual income, it may also be sold in terms of deferred gifts after the initial group has been started. It is critical that the total gift and time span should raise the sights of both board members and contributors and yet offer a realistic goal."[4]

Another method of stimulating annual gifts that is almost as familiar to hospitals as the "Dear Friend" fund-raising letter is the

special event or benefit, designed as a fund-raising instrument but
equally valuable, and in some cases more so, as a means of
publicizing the hospital's good works and engaging the interest
and efforts of dozens—sometimes hundreds—of volunteers who
are thus made to feel they are part of the hospital organization.
The event or benefit has a thousand faces: there are fetes, balls,
garden walks, rummage sales, art exhibits, fashion shows, and
auctions; benefit performances of everything from Shakespeare to
symphony to circuses; exhibition sports events such as golf and
tennis tournaments, horse shows, rodeos, and hockey games;
marathons, telethons, walkathons, bike-athons; feasts, fiestas,
cocktail parties, barbeques. The form of the benefit is a product of
the imagination of the sponsors and the culture of the community.
Long Island's horse show is Arizona's barbeque; California's golf
match is Minnesota's snowmobile rally. Whatever the vehicle, the
success of a benefit is measured in attendance, publicity, net income, and fun.

For reasons that are embedded deeply in the society but show
signs of coming loose in our time, the hospital benefit in the past
has commonly been considered the province of the auxiliary,
predominantly a female phenomenon, rather than that of the
male-dominated board of trustees. The logic of this arrangement is
derivative: The serious business of management was for men;
women could be trusted to handle matters of entertainments. For
all the latter-day inroads on territoriality, the arrangement remains
for the most part undisturbed. The women run the benefits; the
men spend the proceeds.

At times the proceeds may mount to millions. With its network
of community guilds and societies throughout the area, for example, the Children's Hospital of Los Angeles has elevated this kind
of fund raising to the level of an art form. The guilds run shops,
stage bazaars, sponsor benefits, exploit celebrities, make
money—and the hospital depends heavily on this income for its
patient care, building, and special facility and program needs.
Elsewhere, hospital gift shops, snack bars, and other income-
producing enterprises are common auxiliary activities, as are off-
premise white elephant shops, handcraft sales, auctions, and a
variety of businesses that earn for U.S. hospitals several hundred

million dollars a year. And all this is what the auxiliaries do with their left hand, so to speak, while the right hand is busy with the principal auxiliary task of recruiting and deploying volunteers to staff hospital floors, lobbies, offices, and departments and save the nation more hundreds of millions annually. Contemplating these figures, one is constrained to consider that a society clinging to its men-at-the-office-women-at-home traditions was missing something that probably couldn't be discovered by insisting that everybody should go around saying chairperson. The recent rapid rise in the number of women in the work force suggests that the tradition is fading, and it may make its last stand in hospital board-rooms.

CHAPTER 5

The Development Business

For some hospitals, the annual gift campaign is the whole of the institution's fund-raising effort except at times when an intensive drive for a specific capital project is in progress. Others maintain a continuing or recurring program of soliciting major gifts but make no particular effort to encourage annual contributions. In many institutions, however, annual giving is part of an overarching development concept aimed at evoking lasting support for the total hospital enterprise. The annual gift campaign generates funds for current needs and names for future cultivation. On a different level, the development program comprehends the institutional mission over time and seeks to anticipate needs and make certain that support is at hand as the needs emerge. It is fund raising writ large.

In some institutions, and especially in universities, where the concept originated, the development officer is at the top executive level, taking part in the planning and definition, as well as the interpretation and support, of the institutional mission. This is increasingly the case in hospitals, though it is true that in many cases the title has been adopted because it has become the fashion, but the function remains one of providing needed staff support and technical expertise to guide the fund-raising efforts of the trustees and administrators. Inevitably, if not always logically, the more successful the fund raising is, the more likely its practitioners are to be elevated to the institutional policy level.

Wherever it fits into the organization chart, the development program includes a variety of functions and activities. Gonser, Gerber, Tinker, and Stuhr, the educational consultants, have described these: "From our experience in development, we have found there are four phases in obtaining financial support that should be part of a development effort. All four phases should be carried on simultaneously: (1) Annual giving from a broad constituency to undergird the education program. (2) The effort to seek out prospects with special interests who may aid in various projects through grants in moderate amounts or who will build personal funds for special or general purposes of the institution. (3) Bringing major capital objectives to fruition by cultivating those prospects able to provide the large grants necessary for such purposes. From time to time this may involve an intensive solicitation effort for a single capital project. (4) Showing all publics how they can, through a sound deferred-giving program, invest in the blueprint of the institution."[1]

Given an institution and program that can be shown to be needed and worthy, development officers and fund-raising consultants are all agreed that the foundation on which all types of fund raising rests is research that produces extensive and reliable information about who has the money to give and what can be found out about each prospect that will help to determine (1) how much to ask for, (2) what purposes or projects are most likely to evoke the desired response, and (3) who is the best person to approach the prospect and ask for the gift.

Trustees, physicians, and auxiliary members are often sources for much of this information, but they have to be asked for it systematically, and sometimes repeatedly, and often they have to be persuaded that it is necessary for the purposes of the institution to tell what they know about their friends, associates, and patients. Physicians, especially, may consider that an ethical question may be involved, although in most cases it seems likely that a lot of useful information known to the physician can be disclosed without touching on the kind of medical, personal, or family matters that should be regarded as confidential.

Hospitals that have their own foundations or fund-raising committees, separate from the board of trustees, may choose members

of these groups as much for their knowledge of fund-raising op-
portunites as for their ability to solicit gifts, so these groups, too,
can contribute to the stockpile of information about where the
money is. In rural areas and small communities, particularly, these
inside sources may be able to provide all the information of this
kind that is needed; in larger cities, the task may be much more
complicated, but there are other resources.

The resources in common use among development officers and
fund raisers include the directories published by Dun and
Bradstreet, Moody's Investors Service, Standard and Poor's, and
others; *Who's Who* volumes for various areas and industries; the
Foundation Directory and supplements published by the Foundation Center in New York; club and society membership lists; and
newspaper files. Development officers also keep lists of donors to
other institutions and causes whenever these are available, and
many of them also design special mailings for trust officers, estate
planners, lawyers, investment counselors, and others who may be
in a position to advise their clients about gift opportunities. Often
these advisers may pass the word on to an interested client who is
not identified unless or until he wants more information about an
institutional program.

Once the prospects and their potential for giving are known, the
next step is what development people, along with salesmen of
everything from bandages to bridges, call *cultivation,* or as
Carryl Ziettlow of Iowa Methodist Medical Center describes it,
somewhat more delicately, "a process of further identification, an
attempt to find that connecting link of common interest and concern." Actually, it is a carefully planned education, he explained,
"whereby we expose people to the general program of the hospital
in order to particularize their interest. This may include emphasis
on our role as an extension of the healing ministry of the church,
our concern for the child, our rehabilitation programs for accident
or stroke victims or the aged, our training programs for nursing
students, our ability to give special quality to health care for patients because of specific major gifts that resulted in buildings and
specialized equipment. We involve the prospect with key people at
our institution. The executive vice-president is so familiar with the
total operation that he can talk effectively with anyone. If interest

is expressed in a specific area, we try to involve someone there. The individual health care specialist usually is pleased to show and explain the work, and this enthusiasm is exciting. We believe in involving the donor in an emotional way, showing how he or she can extend a humanitarian concern and become an integral part of our healing team through a gift to the institution.''

In the case of great expectations involving a family of substantial wealth, the cultivation process may take on the logistics and strategy of a military engagement. Jack Herman, former vice-president for development at Mount Sinai Medical Center in New York who is now at the Hospital for Joint Diseases there, told about one such case. "In the $150 million campaign, one family contributed $8 million, which was eventually increased to $12 million, to name a building in memory of the mother," he related. "I don't need to point out that such a gift does not come out of the blue. The mother had been a frequent patient at Mount Sinai. The family had a long record of giving to Mount Sinai and had been receiving our annual reports for years. They were familiar with our goals and objectives, were invited to all our important events and dedications, and had received our campaign and major gift brochures spelling out the various projects available for memorialization. The mother's illness coincided with Mount Sinai's plans to build a medical school that would be a major landmark building in New York. So there were many conditions conducive to giving a large amount. The only thing that was missing was the inclusion of the family physician, who was on our staff, to help move the effort along.''[2]

It was the responsibility of the development director to make the necessary arrangements, or to see that they were made, Herman said, "to bring together in as cordial an atmosphere as possible the members of the family, the key person to ask for the gift, and the supporting or backup people such as the family doctor, the administrator, and the development director. It is usually best to keep the group small and intimate. In this case we brought with us an architect's rendering and specifications for the proposed building and pertinent documents to show what the government was prepared to contribute. Our material called for a leading gift of $8 million to name the building. This would also be considered a leadoff gift to encourage others to name lesser parts such as floors and major facilities. This was also done to assure the family that they would not be alone in funding a program as vast as this one was. In reality, it was a push-pull situation involving the federal government, the state, the city, trustees, and other major benefactors in the private sector. When the actual day of the solicitation arrived, all the materials were assembled, everyone knew his role, and the family came forward voluntarily with their gift. The rest of the campaign flowed from there. It was truly a partnership of government and philanthropy, with the private sector giving 65 percent and the government 35 percent.''

Whether the expected gift is $8 million or $8,000, development people all agree with Herman that it is worthwhile to get the prospective donor to visit the hospital and meet with the principals to engage interest and bring the gift opportunities into focus. Another seasoned fund raiser had another suggestion for accomplishing this important strategic objective. ''People will get involved most comfortably in the institutions we serve when we ask them to do something they are familiar with,'' said William F. Hobbie, vice-president of Brakeley, John Price Jones, Inc., a fund-raising consultant firm. ''Asking for such help is probably the best form of cultivation we can employ. Look for places where you can use real help. Are there needs in building maintenance, publications, landscape and grounds, financial planning, public events, volunteer services, security? These are some of the more obvious ways of involving and cultivating. I think boards of trustees could make much greater use of such talents by inviting qualified citizens to serve on special committees and task forces— even on trustee committees—on a short-term basis. This involvement is the best kind of cultivation.''[3]

Cultivation is obviously an extended and painstaking process, and many practitioners consider that it never ends, actually, but should be continued after the gift is made—on the sound principle that there's always more where that came from. But there comes a time when the cultivation process has to be interrupted, or at least supplemented, for long enough to ask for the gift if it hasn't already been offered. Like all development and fund-raising professionals, Hobbie emphasizes the importance of asking for the order, and for those who find it difficult to come right out and ask he proposed this simple formula: "I want to tell you why I am working for Memorial Hospital and believe in it as strongly as I do. I want to tell you why I am giving to it to the maximum I am able to afford. I'll be very frank and warn you that my purpose in meeting with you is to get you to know, and to believe, and to work for, and to give to the hospital, exactly as I do."

When it comes to either cultivation or solicitation, Hobbie concluded, "having the right volunteer leader explain why he or she believes in, works hard for, and gives generously to your hospital is the most persuasive process ever invented." Like most professional fund-raising and development people, Hobbie believes the consultants and staff should organize and arrange and advise and monitor and evaluate, but not actually solicit. At Children's Hospital of Los Angeles, for example, Marti Slosson, the development director, may sit in on the meeting when a donor comes to the hospital and take some part in "the usual arts and graces of continuing cultivation." But she believes the staff for the most part should be anonymous. "Volunteers, peers, do the soliciting," she said, "and the volunteer has to give first."[4]

Certainly that is the prevailing wisdom in the fund-raising culture, but there are notable exceptions. At Memorial Hospital Medical Center of Long Beach, California, for example, development director Eleanor Heldt told about an 80-year-old woman who had been giving the hospital $3,000 a year in memory of her husband. "I enter the picture about four years ago," Heldt said, "and I kept meeting with her and going to see her in her home. In many of our conversations I sensed a need for her to do something a great deal more for her husband's memory. She talked about him all the time, and it occurred to me that an endowment fund for education might be established in his name. We had a new department of education just at that time that needed money to do an overall education job for the hospital: educating patients and staff, and upgrading employees who couldn't speak English so they could relate better to patients and understand orders better. So I told our donor what I had in mind. 'It will be an endowment fund in your husband's name, and we'll put up a plaque on the wall and have the people in the department meet with you and tell you how the fund will be used to help,' I said. And she really caught fire with the idea that this would be a perpetual thing in memory of her husband."[5]

The endowment fund was established, Heldt said. "I feel that if I'm most effective on a one-to-one basis with a donor, then I can establish an excellent rapport with the donors and have no problem in talking with them. Many times we'll have a board member come up with a prospect. I'll come along on the first visit, and if it works out that way, from that time on I handle it on my own."

Jerry Panas of San Francisco is another fund raiser who doesn't hesitate to solicit donors himself when he feels confident he is the best person to do it and the board or the fund-raising committee agrees. "If you're working in a situation and the people who are involved know you, and you've had a good relationship with the board and they respect you as a person and as a professional, there's every reason to feel that you can do a good job of explaining the need for a donor to make a leading gift," Panas explained, "then as an outsider it's possible for you to say, 'I've got nothing personally invested in your project. It's your program, your hospital, and if you really believe in it, this is what you've got to do.' It's very easy to say that on some occasions. There are times when the volunteers are enthusiastic about the project, excited about it, committed to it, and are willing to make the calls, but they simply don't know how to ask for the order, you know? After all, these are amateurs, and so we find that very often it helps to have one of our group go along, so that we can ask for the order."[6]

Panas remembered an instance when a prospect had made a substantial gift that didn't come up to the expectation of what he was capable of doing. "This fellow was devoted to the institution, loved it, and had been involved in it for a long time," he recalled. "When he sent in his gift, it was the result of his enthusiasm for the program, but he just had no idea where he ought to be aiming; he thought it would be considered a major, leading contribution. Well, it wasn't, not in terms of what he could do or what we had in mind for him to do. So as we talked about who ought to make the call on him to lead him to where he ought to be, the board felt that it would be proper for me to do that, because I had been working with him on one of the committees and we had a fairly good relationship, and there was no one else who wanted to tackle him.

"So we talked, and it wasn't a case of trying to convince him of the worth of the institution, because he believed in it. And it wasn't a case of salesmanship. It was a case of bringing to a person who was devoted to an organization a sense of what his responsibility was as one who was committed to the institution and its work and its mission. It was an easy thing for me to do. In the case of each major donor you try to determine what is the best strategy. For some donors it's clearly best for us to stay in the background, as if we didn't exist, and in some cases it's best for us to be involved with one of the volunteers in making the call. Then there are cases where we do it ourselves. And often, as in this case, there are times when a volunteer has called and the gift came in at the wrong level, and as objective outsiders we're able to go to the person and say, 'What you've done I'm sure is the result of a great deal of thought and consideration, but let me tell you what I hope you will consider if this institution is to become what I know you want it to be.' It's that kind of an approach that can make a person jump to a different level, and we've done it time and time again."

In addition to the annual gift effort and the continuing quest for the donor with the pot of gold, every development program is also engaged in seeking out those who may not be ready to hand over cash or negotiable securities or the family jewels but who may be persuaded nevertheless to make some firm commitment making the institution a beneficiary at some future time. According to Weston L. Bonney, president of the Cape Ann Bank & Trust Company, Gloucester, Massachusetts, and also chairman of the development committee and member of the board of trustees at the Addison Gilbert Hospital at Gloucester, such commitments, which are commonly known as deferred giving, can be defined simply as gifts that are legally established during the donor's lifetime but are not received by the institution for its use until some future date. "Examples of common deferred gifts include bequests under wills, unitrusts, annuity trusts, gift annuities, life insurance, and real property with an interest retained by the donor or a named beneficiary until a future date,'' Bonney explained.[7]

Every hospital board with an interest in any kind of fund raising has at one time or another thought to encourage its own members and donors to remember the hospital in their wills. In recent years many have followed the initiative of the colleges that began years ago to establish life insurance or annuity policies with the college as beneficiary. In the past several years, changes in tax laws, among other reasons, have had the effect of multiplying the kinds of deferred giving that may offer positive advantages to the donor, and the result has been that colleges and hospitals now make deferred giving an important component of their development programs. Universities and large medical centers may have whole staffs that spend all their time consulting with donors and prospective donors about their estates, shaping plans that will result ultimately in the transfer of substantial assets to the institutions.

This practice is now being extended to smaller hospitals that may not have estate planning experts on the staff but offer the service through consultants. The Addison Gilbert Hospital at Gloucester, for instance, is a 150-bed institution that first became seriously interested in deferred giving a few years ago when a member of the development committee told about another institution's pooled income fund that had resulted in a major deferred gift to the institution with a distinct tax advantage to the donor. "This example stimulated the committee's interest," said Bonney. "If everyone benefits, it must be a concept that could be sold to other potential donors." To investigate the possibilities, the committee appointed a subcommittee that included two local attorneys who were active in drawing wills and establishing trusts, an accountant, a trust officer, and a business executive, as well as the hospital administrator, the development director, and several members of the development committee of the board. "Based on the knowledge and experience of these members of the subcommittee, it was determined that there was certainly a potential for deferred giving in the community if a way to interest and motivate potential donors could be found," said Bonney. "It was apparent that something more than brochures mailed to prospective donors was needed. The idea of some 'soft-sell' seminars to interest friends and prospective donors in the concept of making deferred gifts where circumstances are favorable was considered.'' Eventually, the hospital retained a consultant to help plan the seminars, and the program was launched.

As it turned out, the seminars proved to be so popular that in order to accommodate all who signed up two sessions were held on each of three topics: wills, trusts, and charitable remainder trusts. ''Many people needed to be reminded to review their financial plans and draw their wills,'' Bonney said. ''The seminars provided a service by stimulating them to do so and telling them how to go about getting the necessary professional help to carry out their desires. Of course, it was hoped that the hospital would be given any favorable consideration in the financial plans of its constituency. We emphasized that their attorneys and accountants should be directly responsible for finalizing plans and drawing definitive instruments, but the offer of help from the hospital development office was made, and we arranged to have our consultant available for professional assistance.''

The consultant was Terry Mayo, who had established his estate planning consulting business after spending several years as a university development officer. Mayo estimated that less than 5 percent of people with estates that need planning have ever done any estate planning. ''If we are going to reach these estate owners,'' he said, ''we must do more than send out newsletters and brochures that decree some fantastic tax-saving idea the content of which doesn't realistically begin to fit either our needs or theirs. If 7 out of 10 people who die don't even have a will, how on earth are we, as development officers, going to convince them to establish, say, a charitable remainder unitrust with our institutions? Let's give the donors, the doctors, the volunteers, the citizens who represent our constituencies an education about estate planning.''[8]

What is needed is a program that will give people the information they need but don't know where to get, Mayo said. Even those who have attorneys specializing in tax law aren't always likely to get the kind of education that is most helpful to them, he suggested. "The tax attorney can write a will or a trust. Maybe he'll do an estate analysis, but he isn't going to explain, for example, the relationship between taxes, ownership of property, and probate unless you are astute enough to ask the question in the first place. So where does anyone go to get information on estate planning? A trust officer? Perhaps, but again, the trust officer is primarily interested in managing estates, not in educating the public. So why doesn't your institution offer such a program as an extension of your ongoing educational services? Many of your organizations offer prenatal courses and conduct programs for rescue squad leaders. Why isn't the offering of informative sessions on estate planning also a service to those you serve in the community?"

The estate planning seminars were the beginning, not the end, of the deferred giving program at the Addison Gilbert Hospital, Mayo explained. There are also written materials focused on Massachusetts estate tax rates and Massachusetts probate law, and, most important, personal follow-up sessions with those who request them. "Here the prospect discusses his particular situation and an attempt is made to assist—not in a legal sense—to the extent possible. We don't write wills or trusts," Mayo added. "But we do read wills and trusts and explain them if requested and discuss contemplated changes. We will do an estate analysis if warranted that shows what the various tax implications are under the present plan, then compare that with options that would include charitable gifts in one form or another. Of course, anyone who requests deferred giving literature, attends the seminars, or receives a personal session falls into a prospect file that is used for ongoing cultivation."

The deferred giving services of Addison Gilbert Hospital are unusual only because of the relatively small size of the institution. University and teaching hospitals frequently offer these and other personalized services. Iowa Methodist Medical Center subscribes to a quarterly financial guide service called "Amicus" for a select group of very important people and, when their interest in the institution is apparent, follows up with detailed information about annuity, charitable remainder trust, pooled income, and life estate contract gift opportunities.

Often consulting services are provided by members of the hospital's own development staff. The Memorial Sloan-Kettering Cancer Center in New York, for example, has a director of income trusts and bequests in the office of the vice-president for development and public affairs. One of many deferred giving programs at Memorial Center is the Robert Hixon Pooled Income Fund, a type of charitable remainder trust established in honor of a well-known leader in the securities business who died of cancer. Through the fund, "a donor can provide long-range support for the center's future and at the same time realize present tax benefits and preserve income to meet family or personal needs by making a capital gift, while retaining the right to income for life for himself or his designated beneficiaries," says a fund brochure. Gifts of $1,000 or more may be dedicated to particular uses specified by the donor, it is explained, or they may be used at the discretion of the trustees. In any event, the income will be paid in accordance with the donor's instructions until the death of the last surviving beneficiary, at which time a principal sum equal to the value of the units assigned to that income interest will be transferred from the fund and turned over to the center. The brochure also explains the income tax, capital gains tax, gift tax, and estate tax advantages and limitations accruing to the donor through participation in the fund, and cautions that "there can be no assurance that particular investment results will be achieved. The income received by the fund and the value of securities and other property held by it will fluctuate with changes in market and economic conditions. The investments of the fund will be diversified and may include both equity and debt securities in such proportions as seems advisable from time to time in light of current market and economic conditions, as well as other real and personal property and cash to the extent the trustee deems advisable. There are no limitations or restrictions on the investments of the fund except that it may not acquire or hold any securities the income from which is exempt from federal income tax. However, it is the policy of the fund not to invest in closely held corporations, oil or gas participations, or other speculative forms of investment with a high risk factor." Memorial Center's deferred giving program also offers the interested donor the opportunity to consider a gift to unitrust, annuity trust, gift annuity, or deferred payment annuity options, and detailed information and advice on all these opportunities are offered by the center.

Summarizing the responsibilities in deferred giving for institutional development officers, Jane Stuber, associate director of development at Smith College in Northampton, Massachusetts, said: "Know your constituency, master pertinent facts relating to your program, develop fluency and accuracy in making basic calculations, build an internal structure for your deferred giving program, keep your volunteers informed and enthusiastic, use the services of your institution's attorney, develop an understanding of investment procedures relating to your donors' gifts, assist your donors' advisers whenever you can, keep abreast of changing technical requirements, and work closely with your institution's chief financial officer."[9]

Gonser, Gerber, Tinker, and Stuhr added a practical grace note: "Too often institutions feel that only the very wealthy are prospects for estate planning. Actually, there is some point in just about everyone's estate picture where a charitable institution could and should figure. Elderly persons, for whom financial management is a burden, are prospects for annuity and life income trust plans. Persons with holdings in real property may find that an institution provides a medium for solving difficult estate problems."

Another Massachusetts hospital trustee commented on the trustee's overall responsibility for the development program. "As the trustee on our hospital board responsible for development, I feel that I am in a very important nerve center," said Townsend Hornor, trustee of the Cape Cod Hospital at Hyannis. "On the one hand, I look to the hospital administrator and to my fellow trustees for initiation of programs that will need money in order to be accomplished. As the development chairman, and as a trustee, I pass on those programs and have a substantial opportunity for input as to their validity and shape. At least as much as the other trustees, I feel that my judgment and reputation are on the line when we agree to move ahead with a program, because as development trustee I must go out and sell it. There can be no backing away.

"On the other hand, I look to our development director to take the need for the program and create around it an appropriate campaign to produce the financial support required. His involvement at the trustee development committee level and through the administrative hierarchy will, I hope, have allowed his important inputs and judgment to filter into the program while it was under discussion, so that when he receives the assignment to go to work he is already both informed and committed to the program's support. Any degree of communication and liaison less than that will make his job a great deal more difficult.

"In the overall perspective of making development work, the development trustee is in a sensitive and important spot for another reason: He is a volunteer, an unpaid trustee, outside the chain of staff command, and the most temporary of the players. And yet because of these conditions, he is in the unique position to make things work, to solve problems outside the chain of staff command, to push and pull and wheedle, and to be unreasonable at times if that is the only way to get things moving. While he is there, he can do a great deal, if he understands the opportunities and is willing to move. He can significantly improve communications among administration, trustees, development staff, and community. He can educate others regarding development, its needs and its methods. He can sell the hospital to new groups of supporters. He can sell the medical staff on the need to support their hospital better. But he must do these things without breaking all the china in the cupboard.

"In these times of ever increasing hamstringing of the hospital by cost containment schemes without end, all of which seem to have the bankruptcy of the private health care system as their logical end, the ability of the development resource to raise equity and allow growth to meet the hospital's needs is of unique importance. Only by a really satisfactory blending of effort of administration, development, and trustees can it succeed."[10]

At every institution where funding has always risen to match a vision of greatness, whether it is a hospital, a university, a church, or a symphony, there has been an inspired person whose dreams are catching, and soon there is a corps of men and women similarly inspired and spreading the word, and finally there is an army of believers, and the institution moves. These things don't just hap-

pen. They are made to happen. Along with the vision of greatness
has been a plan, and a program, and objectives, and guidance, and
careful monitoring every step of the way. Great universities and
medical centers have whole staffs that do these things. Many
hospitals have one or two people, at least, with full-time funding
responsibility. In smaller institutions it may be a board committee
or member, or an administrator, or physician, or volunteer. And
there is often an outside consultant or fund-raising counsel doing
all or some of the organizing, watching the details, and measuring
the results. But ask any of these people why some fund-raising efforts succeed and others fail, and you will most likely get a one-
word answer: leadership.

What is it? Certainly leadership is in part a quality of intellect,
and in part of character, and in part the commonly misused term
charisma in its true meaning, which is "divinely gifted or
favored." This is the grace that makes it possible for leaders to in-
fuse others with their love of an institution or cause. Whatever it
is, it can be more easily demonstrated than described, as it was
when Boone Powell was talking to a visitor in his office at Baylor
University Medical Center. "Over the years, we have been fortunate to have gained the confidence of the people in this area, and
they have given us the financial support we've needed to keep
Baylor in the forefront among health care institutions," Powell
told the visitor, who had asked about Baylor's fund-raising
methods. "This business of saying philanthropy is dead is, in my
opinion, 100 percent wrong. For instance, two years ago for the
first time hospitals moved ahead of educational institutions in
total giving.

"People become real close to hospitals when they have loved
ones who are hospitalized, and I think if the hospital itself has the
right kind of feel and the right kind of approach, a lot of these
people can be cultivated for future support. Now of course it
would be the last thing in anyone's mind to approach a patient or a
patient's family while they're ill in the hospital and say anything in
the way of suggesting a donation. They are your guests, and you
don't treat guests that way. You do the best job you can helping
them through this trying period of their lives, and then, maybe
three months or six months later, if you feel it's appropriate, you

might have the principal member of the family for lunch and talk in general terms, showing some of the things that are going on. Usually that's enough. They begin to ask questions, and they begin to feel that they might like to have a part in something so significant for all the people of the area.

"This really is where most of our philanthropy has come from," said Powell, referring to the $100 million, give or take, that has come to Baylor during his tenure as administrator. "We periodically have community fund-raising drives of an intense nature. These always produce, and we always exceed the goal. Our last campaign was two years ago. We had a goal of $4 million, and we raised $7 million, and we were able to complete projects totaling $11 or $12 million. But even though these campaigns are successful, and we only have them once every eight or nine years, depending on what the need is, the real philanthropy—the real volume—comes on a day-in, day-out basis.

"Usually the procedure is like this: The administrative people, maybe with the doctors and in consultation with the trustees, decide that something is needed for the institution, to add to or improve the services—like our center for continuing education. We felt that there was a need for it. We researched it, we documented it, and then we began to think in terms of who might be interested in this. For any such project, we might have five or six or seven people who might be potential major donors. Once we decide who they are, we'll establish priorities: This will be the first person we'll talk to, this will be the second, this will be the third, and so on. Then we go back and consider the first person we're going to. Now, who knows this person? Many times it turns out to be the administrator, because of the time he's spent with these people. Sometimes it's the doctor, or it might be the doctor and the administrator together, or it's some member of the board who can go with the administrator or the doctor.

"These special projects could range anywhere from $5,000, $10,000, or $15,000, or something like that, and when you get into projects of $50,000 or $100,000, or a quarter of a million or a million dollars, then you really want to package the idea. You begin to think in terms of how you're going to market it: whom you are directing this toward and how exactly you go about it. This is what we've done, and you can look around here and see all we have and realize there is no federal money in this place whatsoever and practically no debt on the medical center itself. At times, we've had to do some long-range financing, but I suppose our amortization schedule right now is probably less than $2 a patient day.

"We've been real fortunate," Powell said, possibly over-estimating the part played by luck once he has set his sights on an objective and a donor. "We've tried to operate a good health care institution. We've tried to meet the needs of the people of Dallas and the surrounding area and develop into a medical referral center, and as a result we have been able to attract an outstanding medical staff. We've done this without any highly organized approach to philanthropy. We are just now for the first time taking on this foundation concept which I think is different from anything else we've ever done. I have an open-door policy, and that usually means people can come in, but what it means also is that you can get out and go all over the place, and drop in on nurses' stations, down in the kitchen, over in the engineering department, and up on the patients' floors. And you see the doctors, and you see the nurses, and you drop in on the patients.

"I always have a little list. Usually it's made up of people I know. Or the doctors may call and say, 'I think you ought to get to know these people, and I'll take you up there, or you just drop in.' I do it whether there is any philanthropy potential involved or not, because I enjoy being close to the operation. But as a result, people respond. Maybe only one person out of twenty—a patient, or a member of a family that might be a potential donor. Someplace down the road this person's name will come up, and there will be an opportunity to show them some new development that they may be interested in like the new cancer center, or the new heart center. And I'm just thrilled to show them something like that. This is the way you get their interest, and usually they open the door the rest of the way themselves. They really do. I think I could write a book on the subject."[11]

CHAPTER 6

The Fund-Raising Business

Innocent of the methods used by some fund-raising consultants and client organizations, the father of two children who were pupils at a private school in one of the nation's largest cities a few years ago accepted an invitation to a Sunday luncheon the school gave "to tell a few of our influential parents about our exciting plans for the future." The school at the time was housed in a commodious but aging mansion, and there had been talk about plans for a new building. Correctly, this "influential parent" assumed that the building plans would be the subject for discussion, and that he would be asked to assist in some way. Incorrectly, he envisioned an intimate, private-dining-room chat with the headmaster at which he and a few others would be asked for suggestions and urged to serve on a committee concerned in some way with plans and finances.

Instead, the luncheon was held in a hotel ballroom, and the few influential parents turned out be be a crowd of 150 or more seated at numbered tables—an arrangement, as it developed, that had been as carefully planned as a commando raid, which it resembled in more ways than one. The program began with an illustrated talk by the headmaster featuring the inadequacies, not to say perils to innocent children, of the antiquated existing structure. It concluded with the splendors of the proposed new building, an educational Taj Mahal that had already been planned down to the last desk and overhead projector.

Then the meeting was taken over in a fashion that the unsuspecting father still remembers with amazement, if not horror: "This man the headmaster introduced as 'a former member of our parents' association who is known to most of you,' but who certainly wasn't known to me, got up and said right away that the reason we were all there was to raise money for the new school and we weren't going to leave until we finished the job. He didn't actually say 'Lock the doors!' but he might just as well have, because anybody who got up and walked out at that point would have had to go home and pack up and leave town.

"To start things off, the chairman said several of the people at the luncheon had already announced their intention to make generous contributions, and he wanted to introduce them. So he called their names, one by one, and as each one stood up, in different parts of the room, he told how much they had pledged. The very first one was going to give $250,000, and everybody clapped like mad. There was one at $100,000 and a couple at $50,000, and $25,000, and so on, 8 or 10 of them altogether, with a lot of applause and buzzing after every announcement.

"After that came the countdown. First, the chairman looked down from the dais at the table nearest to him and said, 'Right here at Table One we've got our good friend Danny Fieldson. I'm sure Danny wants to help us build the new school, as we all do— and we know he can afford to. What are you going to do for us, Danny? Stand up and let us hear from you!'

"There was a minute of awful quiet, and then Danny got up and said he guessed he could give $10,000. He got a pretty good hand for that. Then the chairman shuffled some cards he had and called another name at Table One, and another man got up and said he'd give $5,000, and there was more clapping. People in the back of the room were standing up to look and see who else was at that table. But nobody else at Table One stood up, and after a minute or two the chairman said he'd give them a little more time to think it over and then come back to them. Then he went on to Table Two.

"It went on like that, from one table to the next," the influential parent related. "Once or twice when a name was called and the man got up and said he'd give $5,000, say, the chairman would answer back and say, 'From you, Joe, I won't take $5,000; $15,000, at the least.' And one time when that happened the man thought for a minute and then said 'Ten?' kind of timidly. And the chairman said, 'I'll take it!' and everybody laughed and clapped hard."

When the meeting finally ended, the young father concluded, those who hadn't spoken up when their tables were being canvassed had to line up at another table at the door going out, where they were given pledge cards and their names were checked off a list. Thus the pressure was still on, he said, and he ended up promising to contribute $1,000 over a period of three years. "If anybody had asked me before that luncheon to give $1,000 for the new school building, I'd have said I'd have a hard time giving $100," he concluded.

The method is obviously effective, and it is not uncommon, especially in Jewish charities, according to a British writer, Ben Whitaker. "As in much philanthropy," Whitaker wrote, "the wish for status plays some part. Although the strict Jewish tenet is that charity should be anonymous, the numerous plaques on buildings donated in Israel show that this idea is honored more in the breach than in its observance. A trustee in New York described one method which contributed to this success: 'It was really a type of blackmail. It is still used today in a great deal of fund raising, but it is most open in the Jewish world. Someone will invite all the Jewish businessmen from a particular industry in a city to the Waldorf, and say, "I've got a chart and I know where everyone's sitting, and I know how much you are making." And that's how they raise funds for the United Jewish Appeal and so forth. It's called a card-calling dinner, because when your card is called you have to say how much you're giving. Of course, other denominations do this kind of thing as well, but they're not as open about it. I admire the Jews for being so honest.' "[1]

Not many hospital capital fund drives are conducted by this card-calling technique, perhaps, and yet the method, crude as it may appear to be, simply depends for its effectiveness on a few principles that nearly all professional fund raisers agree are essential for the success of any intensive fund-raising effort:

1. The *need* must be evident and the *case* for the institution made demonstrably clear to the constituency from which contributions will be sought. For a compelling case, you can't beat telling potential givers that their children may be spending their days in a dangerous firetrap you are proposing to replace.
2. The *capability* of the community to contribute the amount sought must be known. It's hard to imagine any closer knowledge of donor capability than the kind that enables the fund-raising chairman to turn down a $5,000 gift because he knows the donor is good for $10,000.
3. Competent *leadership* must be recruited and prepared for the assignment. This quality is difficult to define, but in most communities not hard to identify. Again, the result in the private school case seemed to suggest that it had been accurately identified and successfully prepared.
4. Willing and effective *volunteers* must be found and put to work. Everybody in the fund-raising business will tell you that a volunteer must give generously himself in order to ask for and get generous gifts. In the card-calling method, it's all done in Macy's window.

Another essential that is rarely mentioned in the promotional literature of the fund-raising firms but is always present in one way or another, as it was painfully and obtrusively present at the school fund-raising luncheon, is peer pressure. In most cases, this develops from a knowledge of the community that permits the hospital board or fund-raising committee to assign the task of approaching potentially large donors to volunteers they'll find it impossible, or embarrassing, to refuse. "If I've just made a large gift to your college or church campaign, you're going to have a hard time turning me down when I call on you for a contribution to my hospital," a board member explained, describing peer pressure in what is probably its most common form.

Peer pressure is also at work in donor appreciation dinners and plaques and publications, and it is never out of the minds of fundraising or development professionals as they make their plans and line up their committees. "Fifteen years ago we looked for cheerleader types," Jerold Panas of San Francisco said in reply to a question about the staff of his fund-raising firm, "people who could lead the groups and get them excited. But we don't look for that kind of talent any more as much as we do for those with skills in thinking and planning strategies—how to capture the top 10 gifts and make them fall into place, how to recruit leadership. Before we start a campaign we spend a lot of time trying to determine who are the real leaders in the community, because they're not always the most obvious ones. There are maybe four or five influence groups in any community today, and they are likely to overlap. So what you do is make these little sociograms to determine who these people are and how to get them involved. Finding somebody who knows a great deal about motivating and leading and getting people to do more than they ever thought they were going to do—that takes a special kind of skill."

The combination of what Panas called cheerleader types and the analytic intelligence and skill required to make sociograms is rare, but it may be as good a way as any to describe what it takes to make a great fund raiser, and the quality is probably not much different from that which distinguishes leaders in any field. Great fund raisers might have been great salesmen, great politicians, great generals, or great preachers. In fact, many of the early fund raisers were clergymen who were successful in raising money to build their own churches, then started helping others with their building funds, and eventually branched out into other fields and conducted drives to build colleges, hospitals, YMCAs, and museums. Frederick Gates, for example, who became the principal adviser for the charities of John D. Rockefeller and drew the blueprint for creation of the Rockfeller Foundation, was originally a Baptist minister, and many of the 30 firms in the American Association of Fund-Raising Counsel, Inc., were founded or had predecessor organizations that were founded by clergymen.

One of these, Haney Associates, Inc., of Concord, Massachusetts, got started in the early 1920s when Charles A. Haney, a minister gifted with the same blend of evangelical fervor and business sense that Rockefeller found in Gates, conducted his first campaign for a hospital in New England. Now managed by his sons William R. and Charles Jr., the firm has offices in the South, Midwest, and West Coast areas, and offers fund-raising, development, public relations, and financial management services to hospitals, colleges, churches, and other charitable organizations and institutions. But some of the religious flavor that characterized Dr. Haney's approach to fund raising is still discernible in the Haney emphasis on building community goodwill for client institutions, as well as raising money for them. Bill Haney, now chairman of the board, remembers making trips with his father as a youngster to run errands and help with the details of campaign offices. His deep conviction that communities must help themselves and solve their own problems, instead of leaning on government for support, unquestionably had its roots in his father's evangelistic zeal.

Some 30 years ago, the chief of staff of a small hospital in North Dakota wrote to Dr. Haney following the successful completion of a drive for half a million dollars for a new building. "Six hundred and fifty people here last evening joined together in singing 'Praise God from Whom All Blessings Flow,' " the doctor wrote. "They sang from the bottom of their hearts, and that music-filled auditorium vibrated with a deep and soul-satisfying thanksgiving. Those voices were singing in gratitude not only to the Giver of all things, but to each other and especially to you, Charles, who have so nobly led and inspired this entire community in the campaign for funds for our hospital."

Last year, a trustee of a hospital wrote to Bill Haney: "Your director's greatest contribution to this community, in my opinion, was not the money raised—20 percent over the goal and still coming in. His contribution was stretching this community's mind to a new level of what it could do for itself, far exceeding anything they had ever done before, plus changing a very negative and controversial public relations image about the hospital into one almost 100 percent positive and supportive."

For all his convictions, however, Bill Haney is not especially optimistic about the outlook for philanthropic funding of hospitals. But he makes a persuasive case for the place of hospital philanthropy in this era of borrowing and government support. "Under some government programs borrowing can be at relatively low apparent interest cost," he has said, "but the time lag between application and receipt of funds can see rises in building costs that more than offset the low rate. Furthermore, such loans are accompanied by closing costs and restrictions that can hobble the development of the institution during the pay-off period. Conventional borrowings can be very expensive indeed. Usually from 2½ to 3 times the amount borrowed must be repaid, and even what is thought of as the painlessness of obtaining the loan can prove to be illusory by the time feasibility studies and the costly ritual prelude to granting the loan is endured."[2]

In contrast, Haney insists, fund-raising costs are comparatively less onerous. "Less can usually be raised than can be borrowed," he acknowledges. "Fund raising does require weeks or months of part-time volunteer effort, and it does cost money to raise money —ranging from about 2½ to as much as 10 percent of the amount raised." But even if most of the cost of a capital project is to be met by borrowing, Haney says, there are compelling reasons for including fund raising in the package:

1. The amount raised significantly reduces the amount to be borrowed.
2. Fund raising provides an equity that improves the bond rating and lowers interest costs.
3. A campaign and its accompanying public relations effort usually result in greater awareness of the institution and its services and thus increases revenues.
4. Fund raising also results in some deferred gifts and bequests unrelated to the specific capital objectives of the campaign.

"The wise board borrows carefully and seeks the cheapest available money for its programs," Haney concludes. If it's going to cost anywhere from 2 to 3 to as much as 10 percent of what we raise to hire fund-raising counsel, and if the board members or volunteers who know the donors best are going to ask for their contributions, "Why can't we do the whole thing ourselves?" board members often ask. "What do we get for the money we pay the fund-raising firm that we couldn't do by ourselves for a lot less?"

It is possible that in some circumstances a board might be able to accomplish as much by itself as it could with the assistance of counsel. If funds are being sought for some special purpose such as a research laboratory or cardiac care unit, and if the board already knows the prospects well enough to identify a few potentially large donors known to be interested in the type of project the funds are to be used for, then the board might indeed get the job done without outside help, especially if the hospital staff includes an experienced development officer who knows how to prepare the kind of presentation that is most likely to evoke a favorable response. But even in these special cases it is possible that outside counsel could help the board reach or exceed its objective in less time, and for most institutions in most intensive campaigns for capital funds there are a number of things that can be done by a fund-raising firm that the hospital organization couldn't do without spending as much or more than the consultants' fee to add the equivalent services to its own resources.

The first thing an outside consultant can contribute is an objective feasibility study to examine the hospital's fund-raising history and the reasons for seeking support for the proposed project, in order to assess the validity and strength of the case for the institution; to determine the community's capabilities for contributing the required amount, considering other demands on its philanthropic resources; to test the availability and effectiveness of the needed volunteer leadership; and to measure the attitude or feeling of community leaders and the general public toward the hospital. The feasibility study will include interviews with members of the hospital organization, selected community leaders, a few potential donors and volunteers, media representatives, and possibly representatives of other philanthropic organizations in the community.

The study may take from two or three weeks to two or three months, depending on the size and nature of the community, and it may result in a recommendation to proceed as planned with the fund-raising campaign, in which case the study itself may be a kind of preparation for the fund-raising effort. Often, however, the recommendation may be to change the appeal, raise or lower the objective, or postpone the campaign, perhaps to allow time for a public relations program to effect change in community attitudes.

In any case, a feasibility study by an outside consultant can always find out things about the hospital's relationship to the community that the hospital organization itself doesn't know and probably couldn't find out. For much the same reasons, the consultant may be able to prepare more effective public relations materials for the fund-raising effort than the hospital's own staff can do; it isn't just a matter of public relations skills, but rather the knowledge of what works best for a specific purpose, gained from working with all kinds of institutions in all kinds of communities. Also, the consultant can usually prepare or help the hospital staff prepare the strongest possible statement of the institution's case for use in special presentations for major gift prospects and interested groups, as well as publicity materials for the media and for general distribution.

Another task the fund-raising consultant performs is building the volunteer organization, working with board members and committees to select leaders for the groups that will handle advance gifts, special gifts, corporate gifts, community organizations, and general solicitations. Fund-raising specialists are also essential for building and reviewing prospect lists, setting specific goals for individuals and groups, scheduling and holding report meetings to monitor progress as the campaign progresses, reading clues to detect weaknesses in the organization, and keeping all the machinery working smoothly.

A typical intensive capital fund campaign might last from three to six months, with activities scheduled for every day of every week, from initial preparation to conclusion. Often the consultant may be retained for a follow-up period to ensure maximum collections on pledges made during the intensive drive. It is doubtful that any but the largest medical center or hospital organizations would be capable of conducting all these activities as effectively as it can be done by people who know how and haven't got anything else to do.

The consultant's fee for these and other services is estimated by the professional man-hours involved and the seniority of the consultant's staff assigned to the project. "Costs of programs vary considerably, depending on the scope of the objective, the size of the constituency, and the length of time required," said a release from Brakeley, John Price Jones, Inc., an old, established fund-raising firm and a member of the American Association of Fund-Raising Counsel. "Experience shows that on major capital programs the average cost is about 5 percent of the goal, including professional fees and campaign expenses." It is a canon of the firms belonging to the association that "member firms do business only on the basis of a specified fee, determined prior to the beginning of the campaign. They will not serve clients on the unprofessional basis of a percentage or commission of the sums raised. They maintain this ethical standard also by not profiting, directly or indirectly, from disbursements for the accounts of clients."

The reasons for disapproval of fees based on a percentage of the amount of money raised in the campaign were explained by John J. Schwartz, president of the association. "A standard percentage fee on an especially large campaign might involve entirely too much compensation for the services provided," he said. "A percentage fee might lead to some reports of unconfirmed commitments. It could lead an unethical counselor into settling for much too small a gift from a prospect who, if carefully cultivated and approached in the best possible way, might donate many times the gift in hand. The fee therefore is specified in advance and agreed on by both parties. Since most of the programs conducted by professional counseling firms are for major goals, the costs are remarkably small."[3]

When professional fund raisers are asked why some campaigns fail to reach their goals, the usual answer is that the leaders who looked so good during the preliminary study turned out to be less effective, or less industrious, than had been expected, or some unforeseen condition had intervened, or "the money just wasn't there." But Jerry Panas had a different answer. "When a campaign fails, it is almost always my fault," he said. "If we've done the study and taken it apart and put it together and done our evaluation and thought it through, by then we ought to know what makes that situation tick. Sometimes it hinges on just one or two people becoming involved or making a gift at a certain level. If we understand that and we still don't make the goal, I don't feel that anyone has failed."

Panas told about one small community on the West Coast where there was one man who obviously was the right person to head the campaign. "We interviewed him, and he wasn't interested," Panas related. "We went back to the client and said, 'Your campaign could be successful if we can get this fellow to lead it, and we'd like a little time to work on him.' So we visited him a second time, and finally he took it on. I felt he always wanted to but needed to be talked into it. The campaign exceeded its goal by 20 percent on the strength of that man's leadership, and I take some credit for that, because in that case I was smart enough to know he was the one we had to have. There are some cases where I blame myself for not being smart enough to know how the thing should have fit together. If you've done a good study you should know everything there is to know about the situation."

On many occasions the experience and expertise of fund-raising counsel also can add muscle to what has often been a disappointing feature of intensive fund-raising campaigns: the corporate gifts division. In fact, corporate giving to charitable causes of all kinds, at a fraction of 1 percent of the pre-tax net for all corporations, is generally considered to fall far short of fulfilling the social responsibility of the business sector, a circumstance that prompted the Commission on Private Philanthropy and Public Needs to make its recommendation that the minimum corporate contribution to charity should be 2 percent of net. Moreover, the commission said that the recommended permanent national commission on private philanthropy should consider additional measures to stimulate corporate giving as one of its priority concerns.

"Although the commission recommendation does not contemplate mandatory corporate charitable contributions," the report said, "it does anticipate increased voluntary activity from the business community as a result of wider disclosure of the amount of corporate charitable giving and numbers of donors." The commission recommended that the Internal Revenue Service should continue to be the agency responsible for the oversight of tax-exempt organizations and that the IRS should publish at the end of each year a statement that would include among other things information respecting corporate giving, which "would indicate the numbers of corporations, their size, their industry classification, the value of charitable contributions made, and the charitable categories in which the contributions are made.'' The commission also referred to another report on corporate giving suggesting that this broader base of information would encompass data respecting ''(1) the mechanisms involved in determining the manner in which a corporation calculates its total giving level, (2) the allocation of the total amount committed to charity among different categories of recipients, (3) the priorities and criteria it applied in selecting specific grantees, and (4) the circumstances which obtain in causing a business entity to commit significant resources to charity in light of responsibilities to distribute earnings to shareholders.''[4]

Of course, some economists, and many shareholders, insist that social responsibilities are the proper and exclusive concern of government and the ''third sector'' and that business should stick to its primary goal of earning profits for its owners. But the view of modern corporate management, for the most part, is that corporations, like individuals, have citizenship duties, and that some concern for the well-being of the society in which the corporation conducts its business is thus appropriately regarded as a corporate obligation. Besides, many managers believe that it is good business for a corporation to be known as a generous supporter of worthwhile institutions and causes in the areas in which its people live and work, and that it is prudent from a long-term operating and profit point of view to help make certain these communities have all the services needed to attract a stable work force and keep workers and their families satisfied with their communities and their lives. This means good schools with good teachers and good hospitals with good doctors, and employers increasingly are taking an active part in institutional affairs. What is needed for the good of hospitals and other philanthropic causes is to make this modern management view more widely known in corporations of all sizes and then to elevate the management concept of what constitutes an appropriate regard for the social responsibility of industry.

Professional fund-raising counsel think they know how to do this better than it has usually been done by others, including most hospital trustees and many development officers, who are inclined to settle for perfunctory calls on corporate executives known personally to trustees and solicitation letters to industries in the hospital's service area. In contrast, the experienced counsel or development officer approaches corporate giving with the same systematic, comprehensive organizational concept that characterizes the entire fund-raising campaign or development effort:

- An inclusive list of corporate prospects is compiled, based on careful research in past performance, contributions to other causes, and management's attitude toward corporate and employee giving.
- A corporate gifts chairman is selected who is known to have the modern view of corporate social responsibility and is well known and respected among top corporation executives in the area.
- Prospects are then "sized" for what are considered to be appropriate amounts for their donations and appropriate goals for employee giving.
- Trustees and other volunteers are matched to corporate decision makers and are armed not only with the information required to make the case for the hospital's objectives but also with detailed data on the number of employees and family members of each corporate prospect's group who have used the hospital's services.
- Records are kept of calls and results, and follow-up calls are scheduled as indicated.

There will always be some managements that don't believe in corporate social responsibility, some tightfisted corporation executives who won't give anything, and probably many who will give only token amounts. But experience has shown that the organized approach will pay off in enough cases to make it well worth the time and effort it takes, and there is evidence that the practice of the professionals will pay greater dividends in the future than it has in the past. According to Denis H. Detzel, director of public policy for McDonald's Corporation, a generous donor to charitable institutions, there is a growing need for significant support from corporations for social programs and the need is increasingly recognized, in part because of increased citizen concern about taxation.

"Inside the corporation, stockholders and external relations executives are stimulating management to rethink their contributions policies and programs," Detzel told a recent workshop for clients of Gonser, Gerber, Tinker, and Stuhr, development counselors. "There is a growing recognition that the contributions budget is, in fact, a corporate resource that should in some way work in harmony with other corporate objectives. Organizations of donors have long been attempting to put some order into the generally chaotic condition of corporate contributions programs." But while there do seem to be signs of change in these directions, Detzel said, "there is certainly no imminent wave. For the foreseeable future, corporate development efforts can and should remain well within the 'who you know' mode. It may, however, be worthwhile to begin to examine some of the issues that a change in this mode would raise within the development function."' The changes Detzel referred to were more emphasis on expertise in the selection of not-for-profit boards; more research in the development function; a more central role for the development professional in the management, administration, and evaluation dimensions of the not-for-profit organization; and a more systematic and efficient method for matching donor and donee communities of interest.

CHAPTER 7

The Foundations Business

Private foundations are the source of an estimated 11 percent of all the money provided by philanthropy for all purposes in the United States today. Until a few short years ago, foundations were generally regarded as mysterious benefactors that distributed subventions in accordance with the whims of princes and their latterday counterparts—the very rich and the heirs and disciples they appointed to preserve the corpus and dispose the return. There was some grumbling about the disposition, always, as there had been ever since the Roman emperors served up bread and circuses to quiet the restive, but rarely any questioning the right of the rich to keep on doing as they pleased with what they had.

At least for the past decade, however, the foundations have been under examination, if not attack, from all sides. Radicals on the left began to make headway with the familiar protest that the foundations existed primarily to perpetuate the influence of foundations and their sponsors. When some of the disciples responded conscientiously with grants aimed at redressing long-standing social and economic imbalances, radicals of the right made headway with the charge that foundations were using their influence for subversive political purposes. The Congress moved in with legislation opening foundation operations to some public review and supervision, and a privately appointed Commission on Foundations and Private Philanthropies was generally supportive, but

criticized foundation management for poor financial performance.[1]

On the heels of the commission report, published in 1970,
another study zeroed in on the big foundations, the 33 with assets
of $100 million or more at the time, and concluded that they were
useful but lacked creativity and vitality and would need continued
outside pressure such as government supervision or, better, "the
ethic of social responsibility of the old establishment and the
militancy of some of the newer forms of expression of social dis-
content," a suggestion that could be expected to leave foundation
critics dissatisfied and foundation executives nervous.[2] More
recently, the Filer Commission on Private Philanthropy and
Public Needs gave the critics a voice (see chapter 2) but no comfort, and while its recommendations for added tax incentives for
givers made soothing reading for the faithful, the Congress was
obviously unimpressed.

Meanwhile, the foundations themselves carry on, and a current
estimate shows them spending $400 or $500 million a year, or
approximately 20 percent of all foundation commitments, on
health activities. In one of the most recent of numerous surveys of
foundations, which obviously have an irresistible fascination for
social research investigators, it was remarked that the decline in
health spending noted elsewhere in philanthropy is not observable
in the foundation sector. "One reason that foundations are not
following the general philanthropic trend away from health giving
may lie in the fact that much of the health spending of these institutions is done by small foundations with purely local or at most
regional interest," said a 1978 report of the Health Policy
Research Group of the Georgetown University School of
Medicine. But while a few of the larger foundations have withdrawn from the field, the group added, several have increased
their health spending, and, on balance, "the large foundation
world may be judged to be at least as involved in health sector activities as it was 10 years ago. In current dollars foundation outlays
maintain a small upward trend, but when adjusted for inflation,
their real contribution is decreasing."[3]

One large foundation that is just as involved in health sector activities as it was 10 years ago is the W. K. Kellogg Foundation of Battle Creek, Michigan, which has been a generous supporter of hospital initiatives for more than 30 years. Over that time, Kellogg interests have expanded from a program of support for small hospitals in the rural Midwest to a broad range of projects in education of hospital administrators and trustees, community medicine and public health, ambulatory care, preventive services, family medicine, holistic medicine, and health education of the public, among other things. Like many of the larger foundations, Kellogg is especially interested in pioneering ventures, often providing funds for projects that need help initially but give promise of becoming self-sustaining. The foundation is scrupulous about evaluating the effectiveness of its own program and communicating results widely enough to make certain that others may learn from program successes—and failures.

At whatever level, there is a difference in how large and small foundations spend their health money. The relatively few large foundations devote 93 percent of their health expenditures to long-range investment activities, which the investigators identified as the administrative structure of the health care delivery system, health manpower, facilities and equipment, technology and biomedical research, and financing mechanisms. In contrast, small foundations spend more than half their funds supporting current services. "A recurring theme of the survey findings is the substantial variation in spending patterns among foundations of different size," the report said, summing up. "The data show that in general the smaller the foundation, the less likely it is to be involved in investment activities and innovative undertakings. Smaller foundations are more likely to underwrite hospital deficits and, when they do act in the investment area, to supply funds for maintenance or expansion of the existing health care system."

In fact, the researchers said in the inevitable critical conclusion, "foundations probably ought to be more inquisitive than tradition has required them to be regarding the source and causes of the hospital deficits they are asked to underwrite. Deficits that were historically attributable to losses on services to indigents may have other causes as well, including poor management and excess capacity. . . . The distribution of foundation funds is in practice a function of personalities, politics, individual experience, and analysis, with the last element playing a typically minor role. On balance, this process may be judged to be not greatly different from that determining the distribution of public funds. It could be concluded that, overall, the disposition of private foundation funds has been made with no less wisdom than that of public funds, and on occasion with considerably more. If smaller, local foundations do not serve as particularly innovative forces in American society, rarely either do local governments and other local public spending authorities. Small organizations should not be censured for failing to tackle social problems which may well lie beyond their grasp.''

Hospitals seeking support for a building or equipment or service may not be as interested in how well the small local foundation is serving as an innovative force in American society as they are in the personalities, politics, and experience that determine the disposition of foundation funds. If the trustees, administrator, and development staff or fund-raising consultant are on the job, they have a well-thumbed copy of *The Foundation Directory,* published by the Foundation Center in New York, and they already know whether or not their project or need falls within, or comes close to, what the foundation considers to be the field of its interest and activity. But they may not know exactly how to proceed in order to avoid wasting time and ensure that their project gets the best possible shot at a fair hearing by foundation decision makers.

There isn't any formula for success. Because personalities and politics *are* involved in foundations just as they are in hospitals, corporations, and families, one man's grant may be another man's gaffe. Some years ago, Dr. Franklin McLean of the division of biological sciences at the University of Chicago was seeking support for National Medical Fellowships, a small nonprofit organization he had formed to help finance graduate medical education for deserving black students. Through a friend, he arranged to speak to a member of the board of directors of the Alfred P. Sloan Foundation, who asked for a letter of explanation and a copy of the organization's latest annual report and assured Dr. McLean that the project would have priority consideration. These were duly sent and acknowledged, but months went by with no further word. Dr. McLean had written the foundation off as a source of help and forgotten it, when out of the blue he got a note suggesting that he stop in at the foundation office the next time he was in New York. As it turned out, what had happened was that Alfred Sloan had picked up a copy of the National Medical Fellowships report, a modest document of a few mimeographed pages, was intrigued by it, and told the foundation director to "have that fellow come in and see me."

He did. Within a few days Dr. McLean had arranged to be in New York, hopeful that he might get a grant of as much as $15,000 or $20,000—as much as anybody could expect for what had seemed a bizarre cause in those pre-civil rights days. They talked at some length, and when Mr. Sloan got around to asking how much he had in mind, Dr. McLean, thinking this might be the chance of a lifetime, drew a deep breath and said, "Fifty thousand dollars." Then he almost fainted when Mr. Sloan asked, "You mean $50,000 a year?" That's how it began, and within a few years the foundation had increased its annual contributions and given National Medical Fellowships more than $1 million.

Obviously, foundation giving as a rule is analytic and systematic, and the Alfred P. Sloan Foundation, like others large and small, follows prescribed routines in evaluating proposals and dispensing funds. But whim is not unknown in the best of them, and most foundation executives have stories to tell not unlike McLean's. For the grant-seeking hospital, however, the only sensible course is to assume that the foundation is governed by rules of procedure, find out what they are, and follow them. "The only foundation approach I can recommend, based on personal experience, is a careful study of the foundation's areas of interest and current funding, followed by letter or phone to see if it is receptive to your project," said Cleone M. Vazquez, development director of Mount Zion Hospital and Medical Center in San Francisco. "To do this, you have to work out a succinct summary of what it is you want, why it is needed and how much it is going to cost."[4] Presumably under these circumstances the foundation that is interested enough to consider the proposition will provide specifications, or at least some clues, as to what should be included in a formal proposal and what form it should take.

In the absence of positive indications to the contrary, a foundation proposal should follow the basic rule of organization that was laid down for an oration in Aristotle's *Rhetoric* and is still good for every form of written communication known to man, with the possible exception of novels and short stories: proposition and proof. "Come to the point at the beginning of your proposal," is the way Vazquez put it. "Don't start out with pages of background and keep what it is you want to do and how much it costs to the end. State at the outset how much you want and what it will be used for." Then, assuming the foundation hasn't specified otherwise, "give it the data it needs to evaluate your institution, the personnel who will be involved, and the need you are presenting or the problem you propose to solve. Keep your proposal short, clear, and to the point. Make sure you document your hospital's tax-exempt status and its fiscal responsibility. Make sure your proposed budget is realistic and appropriate for funding by the foundation. Emphasize what will be accomplished."

Somewhere along the line, if the proposition is going to fly, there is likely to be an interview with foundation program people, and Vazquez has some equally sensible advice for hospital trustees and executives for these formidable occasions: "Have with you someone who has the answers at his fingertips to the most technical of questions—the doctor, technician, or specialist who will be directing the project or using the equipment. Be prepared for the most searching and penetrating questions. You can't hide anything in the long run, so level with the foundation." In the case of family foundations, she added, there may be some kind of personal relationship between the hospital and the family, "and the better someone on your board knows someone in the foundation, the better your chances of being funded."

There are 26,000 private foundations in the United States, only a handful of which can be classified as large by the $100 million definition, so there is a lot of homework to be done by institutions seeking grants before they get to the proposal, or even the exploratory letter stage. But the same rule applies to foundations as to other donors: you don't get it by not asking. Institutions that spend a lot of time and money investigating and exploring foundation grant opportunities may be turned down on any number of inquiries and proposals, for reasons that may have little or nothing to do with the merits of their projects. But that doesn't mean they have been wasting their time or money. Foundations are in business to give away money, and somebody is going to get it. If the hospital has a proposition that lies within the appropriate field of activity, by making an inquiry or proposal the hospital is doing the foundation a service, and not vice versa. If there were no applicants, the foundations would be out of business.

A small number of small foundations may be out of business anyway if the American Institute of Certified Public Accountants (AICPA) can't see its way clear to backing off all the way on a proposed audit guideline that would preclude separate reporting of hospital assets and those of hospital foundations, the discrete corporate entities established within the past half-dozen years by hospital boards of trustees to protect hospital endowment funds and unrestricted gifts from being offset against, and deducted from, Medicaid and other third-party payments. "The accounting profession through the AICPA has developed or considered policies that, while they may be good technical accounting, are highly irresponsible as social policy," explained Henry B. Dunlap, executive director of Los Angeles Children's Hospital. "The adoption of these policies would essentially defeat the motivation for private philanthropy, because the donors would be replacing what is otherwise a public responsibility, and few of them would accept this as adequate motivation."[5]

Actually, even before there was any threat of government infringement of hospital assets, hospital foundations existed as a means of making development a more important and prestigious function and stimulating more and larger gifts. Thus there were hospital foundations before there was Medicaid, but there isn't any question that most of the 300 or so such foundations now known to exist owe their origin to the protective coloration the separation of assets appeared to offer after the government programs started looking around for ways to save money. John Vitello, vice-president for community affairs and development at St. Joseph Hospital in Houston, whose foundation was organized in 1964, listed some of the reasons it was considered a good idea at that time. The separate foundation, it was believed, would:

- Provide an opportunity to get prestigious community leaders involved in hospital affairs, especially those with expertise in finance, trusts, insurance, and real estate, when they might not be willing or able to serve on the hospital board itself.
- Relieve hospital board members of responsibility for fund raising, leaving them more time to devote to other hospital business.
- Provide donors with greater assurance that their gifts would be used as requested—sometimes a problem for religious institutions, when some donors may fear that their gifts would go to the mother house, the bishop, or the archdiocese, instead of the hospital and its patients.
- Separate fund-raising costs from hospital operating costs.
- Remove charitable contributions from the hospital's income statement, eliminating the mingling of charitable gifts and operating revenues.
- Provide a more effective vehicle for the investment of charitable gifts and the management of an endowment program, a deferred gifts program, or an investment portfolio.
- Protect charitable donations from lawsuits against the hospital.
- Stimulate life income gifts.[6]

There may also be objections to the separate foundation, Vitello noted, such as possible conflict between the hospital board and the foundation board, with one or the other seeking to dominate decisions, or the foundation board becoming isolated from the hospital and its activities, and donors becoming confused about the disposition of their gifts. But in most places that tried it, the idea appeared to work well. According to Vitello, "the advantages a separately incorporated hospital foundation offer over the traditional development effort in an era of increasing federal controls over the hospital industry are significant enough to warrant serious consideration by the hospital board."

A respected authority on hospital law went further: "A freestanding incorporated foundation, organized solely for the purpose of assisting the hospital as needed with earnings from capital invested by such a foundation, is going to prove absolutely essential for the financial survival of many heretofore unendowed voluntary hospitals," said William A. Regan, a Los Angeles physician-lawyer and author of books and articles on the legal problems of medicine and medical institutions.[7]

That was before the AICPA got into the act with an exposure draft, or trial balloon, proposing modification of financial reporting procedures as these are set forth in the organization's *Hospital Audit Guide*, a topography of accounting practice venerated like the Old Testament among CPAs. The *Guide* called for combined financial reporting for organizations related to hospitals, if they handled significant resources of the hospital and were under the control of the hospital. These were imprecise terms, subject to varying interpretation. Some hospitals and their auditors combined hospital and foundation resources in their reports, and some didn't. The purpose of the modification was to eliminate these inconsistencies and produce reports uniformly reflecting actual hospital resources. But instead, as many saw it, the modification as proposed would only substitute one set of uncertainties for another. What it said was that "resources handled by an organization separate from the hospital are considered to be resources of the hospital if, in substance, their use or eventual distribution is limited to the hospital by the organization's charter or by other means, or is limited to support activities managed by, or otherwise closely related to, the hospital."[8]

This was intended to mean that foundation resources were to be reported separately or "commingled" with hospital resources according to whether the foundation was uncontrolled or controlled by the hospital. The AICPA said that it would be controlled if the hospital's board or other hospital representatives constituted a majority of the foundation's board, or had the power to appoint or remove a majority of the foundation board, or if hospital representatives on the foundation board had special voting rights. But left up in the air were such matters as the precise meaning of "in substance," "otherwise closely related to," and "by other means." Hospital and foundation directors and lawyers and accountants immediately raised these and other questions, and objected also that in the case of controlled foundations the AICPA held that only donor-restricted funds could be reported separately, whereas uncontrolled foundations could separate funds restricted by the foundation or the donor—a critical distinction in view of the government's attitude toward such funds. "The language of the exposure draft can only perpetuate the chaos in auditing and reporting that the guidelines are apparently intended to correct," said a lawyer who handles tax matters for hospitals and health care organizations.

These criticisms came not only from hospital representatives but also from some AICPA members, who made a particular point of objecting that audit reports following the recommended procedure would mislead rate-setting agencies, payers, lenders, and others by including as hospital resources funds controlled by foundations under trusts, grants, and other conditional agreements and not actually available to the hospitals. Responding to all these criticisms, the AICPA committee responsible for the draft withdrew it for further consideration and amendment. Early redrafts that had only limited circulation were not especially encouraging.* Pending further action, hospital administrators, trustees, and lawyers were juggling the comparative advantages of keeping their controlled foundations at some risk of invasion of unrestricted funds and income, as opposed to organizing clearly uncontrolled foundations, protecting unrestricted funds and offering certain other opportunities but risking the possibility that a "runaway foundation board" might be not only out of control but out of sight.

There are also tax advantages and risks to be considered. The controlled foundation that is expected only to raise money and

---

*A revised exposure draft circulated by the committee in September 1979 explained how a hospital might have the ability to direct the management and policies of a related organization without having a majority vote on its board, and thus the related organization would still be considered controlled by the hospital for purposes of financial reporting. The revised draft also said the hospital would be considered the sole beneficiary of the related organization if the latter "solicits funds in the name of and with the expressed or implicit approval of the hospital, and substantially all the funds solicited are intended by the contributor, or are otherwise required, to be transferred to the hospital or used at its discretion or direction."[9] Other conditions under which the hospital would be considered the sole beneficiary were if it transferred some of its resources to a related organization whose resources were held for the benefit of the hospital, or assigned certain of its functions, such as the operation of a staff residence, to the related organization. But it still wasn't clear whether the AICPA would require combined financial statements unless the hospital met both the control and sole beneficiary conditions, or whether separate statements would be acceptable in either case.

make grants can easily qualify for tax exemption along with the hospital, but the uncontrolled or independent foundation that may also own and operate a medical office building or undertake to sell goods and services to the hospital and others must either pay taxes like any other corporation or seek public charity status under other provisions of the Internal Revenue Code. The problems are complex and often recondite and can be resolved only by individual institutions, working with their attorneys and tax consultants.

There may be disagreement always as to which course is best, but attorneys who advise their clients about independent foundations agree that the composition of the foundation board is all important. "Don't play games with it," warned John J. Whitney of the Cleveland firm of Ford, Whitney, Crump & Schulz, who has represented hospitals, colleges, and universities and comes down on the side of the independent foundation. "Hospitals would prefer to control the foundation and use all its funds, but that kind of corporate structure won't do what needs to be done to shield external funds," he advised a meeting of hospital executives. But it is unwise to try to keep effective control by having only the bare legal majority of board members who are not hospital representatives, he added. "Make it genuinely independent: 3 out of 15 board members, say, not 4 out of 6. And don't have all the meetings at the hospital. Respect the ground rules for tax exemption." Whitney believes the independently organized foundation can be "an enormously valuable tool for conserving and enhancing hospital revenues," and he discounts the risk of runaway foundations. "There's no reason to believe the foundation will become any different from a friendly contributor, if the hospital is doing its job," he said.[10]

Sherwin Memel of Memel, Jacobs, Pierno & Gersh, Los Angeles, envisions the independent public foundation as the principal vehicle for a thoroughgoing reorganization of the hospital corporate structure, with separate entities conducting the three main types of activity—health care delivery, management, and investment—that he thinks are going to be necessary to meet the challenges hospitals will face in the future. "The reorganization should enhance the ability of the family of entities to carry on these three separate but related activities in order to accomplish the goals of a financially successful hospital that is a leader in providing cost-effective, high-quality health care," he said.

"The trick is to reconcile the need for separate entities with the need to maintain a relationship among them," Memel suggested. "Given the vagueness of reimbursement rules concerning related organizations and the uncertainty as to the exact nature of future regulatory programs, it is difficult to achieve both the requisite independence and unity of purpose," he explained. But there are a number of measures he thinks could be taken in an attempt to do both things at once. "The management company could be owned by the foundation. While the hospital would be a separate entity, it could be managed by the management company. There could be some continuity of relationship between the hospital's governing board and the foundation's through a limited number of common members. All activities of an investment nature should flow to a foundation divorced from hospital operations. This will help to insulate surplus revenue from spend-down requirements and give donors and management flexibility in using donations."

If he had thought of it when he was organizing and selling his capital stock plan to create the Pennsylvania Hospital in 1751, Benjamin Franklin would have applauded the Memel concept—and made it work.

CHAPTER 8

The Public Relations Business

One of this country's celebrated scholars in the field of linguistics
lectures and writes frequently about the difficulty all of us have
saying precisely what we mean, and then, when we have managed
to do that, how much more difficult it is for us to be understood as
having meant just what we intended to mean and have indeed said.
As an example, he likes to use the simple sentence, "The shooting
of the hunters is terrible," which appears to mean that the hunters
are terrible shooters. But then, he points out, it might also mean
that the fact that the hunters are shooting is terrible. Or it could
mean that the hunters are being shot, and that's terrible. Or that
the people who are shooting the hunters are terrible shooters.*
Then, of course, he goes on to make the point: If a simple
declarative sentence with easily understood, tangible referents can
mean four or five different things, what chance have we got of saying what we mean and understanding one another when we talk
about abstractions like freedom, and democracy, and truth, and
justice, and peace—things we talk about all the time that obviously

---

*I came across this example several years ago in an essay on linguistics in the *New
York Review of Books*. I can't remember now whether the essay was written by
Noam Chomsky, the Massachusetts Institute of Technology professor of
linguistics, or whether it was an essay by somebody else about Chomsky. In any
case, the example is associated with him, and attributed to him here, perhaps with
injustice to an author whose name I don't remember—another common cause of
misunderstanding.

have different meanings for different people? And in this context, what chance do we have of understanding one another when we discuss, as we do right along, such abstractions as health, and health care, and health care delivery? And perhaps the most common of all our abstractions in daily use, *the public* and *public opinion?*

Under the circumstances, it may be foolhardy to write anything on public opinion about health care, especially as it relates to philanthropy, another abstraction subject to varying interpretations. But what we are considering here mainly is hospital care, which is a lot more specific than health care, and mainly giving money to hospitals, which is less abstract than philanthropy. And what is meant here by *the public* and *public opinion* may also become less abstract than is often the case. But it isn't a bad idea ever in considering these abstractions to bear in mind that the ice of understanding is always thin. Consider the public opinion poll, a phenomenon of our time that makes and breaks presidents, influences the composition and disposition of the Congress, starts and ends wars, and is about as abstract as you can get, consisting as it does of how a few hundred people at a particular moment interpret the questions or issues that are presented to them, usually things they haven't thought about one way or another until the question is put, often in ways that suggest an answer, which is promptly given and forgotten—and then reported as public opinion.

The process is so patently fragile that a respected polling organization was constrained recently to explain how it happened that polls taken at the same time had resulted in widely divergent answers on such subjects as the energy crisis, the SALT treaty, and approval of the President's policies and actions. "In view of the sharp disparities that polls can and frequently do show, it seems to us dangerous to let sweeping generalizations get abroad as to what public opinion is," the Roper Organization, Inc., said in a communication to its clients. Commenting on the fact that a Roper poll had shown 66 percent of respondents opposing gasoline rationing while a CBS-*New York Times* poll the same week had 60 percent favoring gas rationing, the communication said, "Small differences between the surveys might be explained by a number of things, including sampling error. A difference of this magnitude can be explained only by a difference in the two questions asked and probably also in part by the context in which they were asked. . . . An analysis of the questions asked in most instances makes the reasons for the very different results that occur clear, and in the process adds perspective and value to the results of any given poll. The danger, however, lies in anyone taking action based on the 'conclusion' cited in the poll report without analyzing the questions asked."[1]

But because few of us have an opportunity to know, much less analyze, either the questions or the context, and fewer still are in a position to take any action based on polls anyway, the real danger may lie in considering that the process, whatever the result, reflects anything that ought to be called public opinion. An example of the phenomenon of particular interest here is the public opinion poll on hospital costs, a topic that has been a lively source of traffic and revenue in the oracle business for the past several years.

Now there can't be any questioning the fact that members of the Congress and the state assemblies, federal and state bureau chiefs and department heads, corporation presidents and union leaders, Blue Cross and insurance executives, and organizers of consumer coalitions *are* exercised, if not panicked, about the rapid rise in the cost of the services they have legislated or are buying or paying or bargaining for, for their constituents in the public programs and their employees or policyholders or members in the private programs. Because it is their problem and their responsibility, they are all constantly making statements and pronouncements about the excessive cost of hospital care and what ought to be done about it, and because of who they are, what they say is reported in the newspapers and on television news broadcasts, and the daily horror headline about hospital costs has become a staple in the news business. So what is the respondent going to say when an interviewer for a public opinion poll comes to the door or calls up and asks what he thinks about hospital costs, or when a questionnaire on the subject shows up in the mail? Unless he just got out of the hospital, it is unlikely that he has ever given the subject more than a fleeting thought. But the question calls the headlines to mind, and he has an instant response: "Terrible! Outrageous! They ought to do something about it!" Because if he says anything else he is going to look like an idiot who doesn't know what is going on in the world. And this "idiot effect" may be multiplied by the wording of the question, as when one recent poll put it this way: "Do you think the health care system is out of control and needs to be changed?" When you call that public opinion, smile.

To the extent that there is such a thing as public opinion about hospitals, it can probably be measured most reliably not by what people may say in response to loaded questions but by the way they behave. This was demonstrated dramatically in the fall of 1977 when the Department of Health, Education, and Welfare's Health Resources Administration published proposed health systems guidelines that recommended closing hospital obstetric departments having fewer than 500 births a year. The same guidelines would have raised questions about the continued operation of any hospital averaging less than 80 percent occupancy. In the first few weeks following publication of the guidelines, HEW got 55,000 letters of protest, and the number eventually exceeded 70,000.

Seeking to find out what happened, HEW picked out two communities whose letters seemed least likely to have been the result of organized letter-writing campaigns, and a consultant was sent to interview people in Sibley, Iowa, and New Braunfels, Texas. What had happened was simply that people were terrified to think that young mothers might have to be driven 40 to 60 miles away from home to have their babies, and the possibility that everybody might have to go that far to get care for sudden illness or accidental injury was seen as a serious threat to both communities. People were fearful of being left without essential protection for their health, and they were infuriated that planners in Washington would try to tell them what they could and could not do about their hospitals. The threat to community health was bad enough, but the insult to community independence and community pride was much worse. By the time the HEW consultant got there, the proposed guidelines had been withdrawn and modified, but the communities were still seething. That's public opinion.

Understandably in today's climate, hospital executives and trustees and their public relations advisers are sensitive about public criticism of hospital costs, hospital management, and occasionally hospital care. It is their responsibility to be aware of such criticisms, to respond appropriately when it is unjustified, and to see that something is done about it when it isn't. Preoccupied with these and other concerns, they are often misled by the headlines and the putative public uproar about hospital and health costs out of control, and they lose sight of the fact that their hospitals could probably count on the same reservoir of good feeling that the people of Sibley and New Braunfels demonstrated when they thought their hospitals were threatened.

City hospitals have an obviously different set of public conditions to deal with. Often their patients come from a diversity of areas, and sometimes the immediate neighbors see the institution as a monolithic menace and a cause of traffic and parking problems, rather than as a comforting resource in times of need. And the institutions may see their neighbors as burdensome troublemakers and unpaid bills, or both. But even huge city hospitals in deprived or low-income areas have seen something of the Sibley-New Braunfels effect on occasion, as in cases of disaster or tie-ups of hospital services due to strikes, when an astonishing number of those troublemakers and unpaid bills have walked in off the streets to offer their services. Everybody knows and appreciates what hospitals do, and that's public opinion, too.

A generation ago, when there weren't any hospital public relations people and fund raising was the primary responsibility of hospital trustees, directed and assisted by fund-raising consultants at times of intensive effort, the institution's only communication with the outside world was an annual report consisting of brief statements by the president of the board, the administrator, the chief of staff, the superintendent of nurses, and the treasurer, and a list of contributors to the annual campaign for the free care fund. Interest of the media was limited to inquiries about accident victims and patients whose names were news; these were handled routinely by the nursing office, or, in rare cases, the administrator. The process was simple because the rule was simple: no comment.

Doctors never spoke to reporters, and in this as in other matters
the hospital was obedient to the traditions of medicine. Publicity
for the fund-raising drive was prepared by the fund raisers, who
produced a brochure with a statement of the case, or need, which
everybody knew about anyway because the need was simple, too:
more room. The fund raisers also called at the newspaper office
with releases and pictures of the proposed new hospital or addition, and the newspaper always published the story or stories—
reluctantly because of the hospital's attitude toward the press, but
necessarily because the biggest names in the community headed the
drive and couldn't be ignored.

All this began to change during World War II and the years that
followed, when scientific knowledge was growing at an ever accelerating rate, new applications in medicine were occurring right
along, hospitals were expanding rapidly and becoming more and
more specialized, newspapers became aware of the widespread interest in medicine, and television began its onslaught on the public
consciousness, with an impact on our lives and our value system
that we still understand only dimly. As a result of all these
developments, the public relations function of the hospital today is
as different from that of the 1930s as a coronary bypass is from a
mustard plaster.

Because everybody knows what hospitals do, the public relations task is first of all one of filling in the details: the range and
nature of the services, the kinds and amounts of skills required,
the technology involved, the changes that are always being planned and carried out to meet new needs for service or simply to keep
up with the advances of medical science, and the whole range of
issues and problems concerning cost and finance. These are the
stockpiles of information and intelligence that need to be sifted,
refined, and packaged in varying ways for trustees, physicians,
employees, patients and families, politicians, business leaders,
community groups, the media, and, of course, donors and prospective donors.

The nature of the hospital mission is such that the public relations people are always busy, too, putting out fires: misunder-
standings or mishaps involving services, problems of billing and

cost and payment and insurance, VIPs who must have handle-with-care attention, accidents, emergencies, cases that involve reporters and require detailed, person-to-person treatment. And on still another level, for selected components of all the audiences an important public relations assignment today is the necessity for improving understanding of the impact of inflation, health legislation and regulation, the advancing technology, and other pressures of the economic, social, and political environment on the individual voluntary hospital and the voluntary hospital system. Continued philanthropic support for the institutions and the system will be needed for them to meet all the demands for public service and at the same time resist all the demands for public control, to survive and remain strong. Thus the tasks of public relations and development or fund raising are interdependent and must be coordinated or integrated if they are to be conducted successfully.

They aren't always that well coordinated, however, and one of the reasons is historical. In most hospitals, the public relations people were already there when the trustees became convinced that fund raising should be a year-round, full-time function, and because the two have to work together and to some extent the jobs require about the same skills, there are jurisdictional questions. The nature of the assignment requires that the development officer work closely with members of the board of trustees, for example, and the public relations director may work mostly with reporters and department heads and never see a trustee except for an interview for the annual report—a contrast that may cause resentment. Or the public relations director may function at a high policy level and consider that the development program is just another department for which materials must be prepared when time permits. Neither of these situations is uncommon, and neither is likely to result in consistently effective performance.

Public relations and development people often argue about how the relationship should work—public relations as a part of development, or development as a part of public relations, or as separate but equal departments. It doesn't really matter, but in any case the management needs to decide which it is to be and make it clear to everybody, and then insist that it should work that way. Effective development in all its phases depends heavily on the production of competently prepared public relations materials, available on schedule, and often in a hurry, as when a hoped-for meeting with a prospective large donor suddenly becomes possible to arrange on short notice and a special presentation must be put together, sometimes overnight. Situations like this are nothing new to hospitals. They happen all the time in the emergency department and on nursing floors, and the public relations and development people have to be just as flexible as the doctors and nurses are, and just as ready to get the necessary jobs done no matter who is imposed on or inconvenienced.

However these activities are conducted, there has been a disposition in recent years for hospitals to refer to some of them as marketing, and the organization of marketing departments, appointment of marketing directors and consultants, development of marketing strategies, and reporting of marketing results have been lively topics for discussion among hospital executives. At every meeting of hospital administrators and trustees there has been at least one scheduled session at which a marketing professor from one of the business schools or a marketing executive from another industry has brought the word to the hospitals, which are presumed to be innocent of any knowledge of the subject. Actually, it isn't anything new to hospitals. For years, most of them have been studying the composition and movement of populations in the areas they serve, recruiting physicians as needed and expanding or adjusting resources accordingly, and through one means or another making their services known in their communities. These activities have usually been described as planning, development, and public relations, not marketing, for the obvious reason that for most people marketing implies promoting and aggressively selling. The principles of medical ethics constrain physicians from soliciting patients, and it has seemed inconsistent for medical institutions to engage in practices that are unacceptable to medicine.

The reason for the surge of interest in marketing has been that, in its anxiety about cost, the federal administration has become convinced that hospitals are overexpanded, and the health systems agencies are determined to "shrink the system" by cutting down what are seen as excessive or unnecessary services. This pressure has heightened competition among hospitals as they seek to avoid being singled out as unneeded, and the marketing geniuses are offering to show them how to "build census constructively," as one of them said, which wasn't exactly what the HSAs had in mind.

Ironically, the interest in marketing, whose function in industry basically is to produce more sales and more profits, has come to the hospital field at precisely the moment when for the first time in history the goal is not more service but less. At about the same time, too, an administrative ruling of the Federal Trade Commission has decreed that the "ban on advertising" by physicians, as the ethical principle prohibiting solicitation of patients was described, was a violation of the antitrust laws and should be discarded so that physicians can advertise their services, like drugstores and supermarkets. The FTC notion was that this would stimulate competition among physicians and bring prices down. But the fact is that in the market for medical services, unlike others, demand is comparatively unaffected by price. The basic determinant of demand is epidemiology—the number of people who get sick or hurt and need services—and epidemiology is not to be manipulated by either price or marketing strategies.

The American Medical Association appealed the FTC ruling and sought to point out that the ethical restraint on soliciting patients is aimed at protecting them from being sold unneeded or inadequate services, thinking they are getting a bargain, and that people are unable to judge the quality of medical service as they do shoes and shaving cream. The same ethical constraints on advertising and soliciting patients apply in the case of hospital services, for the same reasons. There is, and always has been, competition among hospitals, but it has been competition for the kind of excellence that reassures physicians and patients, not the kind of price that allures the unknowing and unwary. And it would be disastrous for hospitals to compete using the marketing tactics of gas stations: "Get your tonsillectomy at St. Swithin's—30% off! This week only!"

Hospitals also compete for donors and donations with other hospitals and with alternative choices of institutions and causes seeking philanthropic support. The public relations component of development, like the public relations component of marketing, is to make the hospital's services for patients and the community known, in this case to prospective contributors as well as to the public at large. The hospital's reputation and prestige are important. In annual campaigns for funds and special fund-raising events such as benefits, the person who gets a letter seeking support for an institution known or believed to have good doctors and good services is more likely to respond with a contibution than he would be to a letter from a place he never heard of. For the same reason, a prospect for a large donation or bequest will be most responsive to the needs of an institution of high professional standing. Public awareness doesn't go to nice professional distinctions, but the task of public relations is to make certain that the professional standing and achievements of the physicians are not regarded as professional secrets. The FTC may not see a difference between this and the advertised cut-price tonsillectomy, but the difference is there, and it is in the public interest to keep it there.

The public relations component of development, however, has to be focused. The annual fund-raising letter usually asks for contributions for a specific service or purpose, and the intensive capital campaign and special donor presentation are likely to be even more explicit, not just because unrestricted gifts may be vulnerable in today's regulated hospital economy but because fund-raising experience suggests that the more focused the appeal, the more likely it is to be successful.

It is in the preparation of such presentations that the integration of development and public relations talents and resources can be most effective. If he has done his homework, the development officer knows a great deal about the interests of the prospective donor and the elements of hospital performance and service and need that are most likely to evoke the sought-after response. Working with the trustee or physician or administrator or volunteer who knows the donor best, the development and public relations people can shape the kind of approach that is called for: the facts of hospital performance and service to be cited, the gaps in facilities or equipment that must be filled, the nature of the service to be offered, the evidence of need, the number and characteristics of the people to be served, the examples, the amount of money that will be required, and the ways it will be spent. And, finally, the kind of presentation to be made: Is this a donor who may be most impressed by an attractively prepared book of text, charts, and tables that he can review with his lawyer or accountant or perhaps other members of the family? Would he be more responsive to a slide film presentation? Or would he regard these as extravagant or unsuitable and prefer a simple memorandum, or perhaps only a conference, with a minimum of supporting documents? And in any case, which of these approaches might be most adaptable for presentations of the same or similar proposals to other prospective donors?

These are not questions with precise answers, but judgment calls, balancing the development officer's desire to cover all the possibilities with the public relations director's love of rhetoric, the administrator's penchant for facts, and the trustee's or volunteer's instinct for what will work best in the particular case. It is a team effort requiring a combination of talent and hard work, and for those who do it best it is also an art form. "It's like a fascinating game," said a young man who is a trustee of a university and a hospital and has been an effective fund raiser for both. "I believe in what the university and the hospital are doing, and I think it's terribly important for them to have the support they need to carry on their work, so the government won't take over any more of it. I'm excited and proud of the part I've had in these institutions, and I get the same kind of thrill and satisfaction from a major donation that I get from a big sale in my own business."

Although public relations considerations are involved in every phase of development and fund raising, the most obvious needs for integration of the two activities, in addition to the preparation of fund-raising letters and special donor presentations, are probably in the publication of the annual report and in planning and preparing publicity for auxiliary activities and events—the annual fashion show, garden walk, debutante ball, or whatever special occasion the auxiliary sponsors on a continuing basis.

The annual report, for example, has come a long way since it consisted entirely of terse official statements and lists and was read by nobody but the officers. In contrast, the hospital report today is the showcase of the public relations effort. Often it is an expertly written, internally consistent exposition of the institution's facilities, services, activities, and plans, generously illustrated and attractively reproduced, with easily grasped and effectively presented statistical and financial information. It is prepared and published not only for the official hospital family—trustees, medical staff, key employees, and auxiliary members—but also for a wide readership among patients and former patients, leaders of business and industry and community affairs, donors and prospective donors. Where there are separate public relations and development departments, copy and layouts for the annual report are usually the responsibility of public relations, with development advising, and the circulation list draws heavily on development resources. Without being too obvious about it, which would diminish its public relations effectiveness, the report is, or can be, a basic and compelling fund-raising instrument, and often the opener for a focused approach to influential donors.

Special events sponsored by the hospital auxiliary are important sources of revenue, in many cases producing hundreds of thousands of dollars for the hospital year after year. They also offer unequaled opportunities to get important people working for the hospital and interested in the hospital, frequently to the point where the workers become significant donors themselves. The events can be a public relations director's dream, combining the news opportunities of the event itself, the important people, the institution, and the patient care services or facilities that will benefit from the proceeds.

The special event is also hard work. Usually auxiliary committees with benefit responsibilities start planning next year's event as soon as this year's is over. They meet often, and often at length, all year long, assigning committee responsibilities, recruiting workers, selecting performers or participants, choosing sites and menus, selling tickets, and organizing all the management details of a big business. Usually there is a public relations or publicity committee working with the hospital public relations department, finding sponsors who are often sources of added revenue, planning and preparing program copy, selling advertising. Through the media people they work with all the time, the public relations staff can help arrange for newspaper and broadcast publicity not only for the event itself but often for many of the preparatory activities, so that the benefit may become a year-round opportunity for publicizing the hospital and the patient care services the benefit is organized to support.

Reflecting on the tandem roles of public relations and development, an executive whose experience covers both functions in hospitals and universities suggested that they are both Johnnies-come-lately to hospitals. "They are adjuncts to the system," said Blossom Porte, now a principal of Health Education Publications, Inc., Chicago, "—added to, but not an essential part of it. Historically, they had a common root, and by comparison with other components of the system, that root is not too deep. . . . The coincidence of a president with polio led to a major involvement of the public with health, and the dimes that marched to conquer that disease are responsible for the billions of public dollars that flowed subsequently into every artery of the medical system. Although it was the overt goal of our professional forebears to garner those goodies, the method adopted was to influence public opinion in more subtle ways—to relate stories of medical miracles, to pull heartstrings by publishing pictures of beautiful children doomed to disease, held in the arms of compassionate nurses. . . . Then we realized that important audiences were also inside, as well as out there. We began to recognize that our potential donors and articulate supporters were seldom the general reader, but often the satisfied and grateful patient. We began to think that employees whose psychic satisfactions matched or exceeded their salaries were as vital to public relations as our typewriters and Xerox® machines, and so we created programs and publications to ingratiate, educate, please, and implore the work force toward that end."

Mrs. Porte has no patience with public relations and development people who worry or quarrel about precedence. "If an assignment must be made on an organizational chart, the decision is most effectively arrived at not on administrative theory but on a practical basis of the people involved," she said. "To be workable and to make a valid contribution to the employing institution, the chart must reflect the talents, interests, personalities, and demonstrable abilities of both individuals. . . . What constitutes a workable, logical interface between public relations and development is the same as it is between administration and medical staff, between nursing and the laboratories, between the social services department and the comptroller's office. It is a bond of understanding, an adherence that gives body to both and strength to the structure it serves. Which piece faces which way is not the critical point. True elegance requires that they be cut of the same mind—a genuine concern that the customer gets what he wants, that the bills get paid, that the deliverers of the product are honest and polite and informed, that the cost be equitable and the product meets established standards."[2]

A seasoned development officer added a word about another vital role. "I'm the coach, not a player," said Tom Dunworth of the Evanston (Illinois) Hospital. "I do the scouting and keep the records and plan the plays, but without active and enthusiastic board members who are willing to give generously themselves and go out and ask others to do likewise, we wouldn't get anywhere."

CHAPTER 9

Asking and Giving Tomorrow

Anybody who is inclined to take a dim view of the future of philanthropy in the United States doesn't have to look around very hard to find the data and authoritative opinion needed to support the position. Total giving has been rising steadily, to be sure; the amount given for all charitable causes doubled in the 1960s, and doubled again in the 1970s. But when the accelerated inflation of the '70s is taken into account, it is plain that giving was slowing down in the past decade, barely keeping up with the inflation in the most recent years. Giving for health and hospitals followed a generally similar pattern, but here the decline was even more noticeable, because total health expenditures were rising rapidly, fueled by the public spending programs. Whereas philanthropy accounted for 6 percent of all health spending in 1966, the year Medicare and Medicaid began, it had shrunk to 3 percent of the total in 1978, not only because Medicare and Medicaid were paying 40 percent of the total hospital bill by that time but also because in the 1970s borrowing had become the leading source of capital for hospitals—on the order of two-thirds of all capital funding, compared to 9 or 10 percent for philanthropy.

These facts cause long faces among the hospital faithful. "Philanthropy will diminish further over time as an influence on the financial operations and capital expansion of hospitals," said

Joseph Terenzio, president of the United Hospital Fund of New York City, one of whose purposes is to promote philanthropic support of the city's voluntary hospitals. Terenzio was speaking at a national conference on capital financing for health facilities, and nobody at the conference disagreed.[1] In fact, the only disagreement among the bankers and investment counselors taking part in the discussion was with Terenzio's conclusion that the decline of philanthropy was a bad thing. It wasn't that they were opposed to giving; they just didn't think it mattered that much any more. "There are places where people don't believe in philanthropy," one of them said. "They think it is unconstitutional, or at least that it has negative connotations."

One place where the negative side gets full play is Washington. "The government is the enemy," said James F. Clarke, who is director of development at the Kettering (Ohio) Medical Center and listens carefully to the negative voices in Washington as former chairman of the National Association for Hospital Development's government affairs committee. "There are people in Washington, including congressional staff and HEW staff, who want to do away with philanthropy," Clarke said. "Their argument goes like this: Part of the contribution given by an individual to a charity is, in effect, public funds. If a donor paying taxes in the 70 percent backet gives $100, he is sacrificing just $30 of his own money, plus $70 that would otherwise have gone to the government. There's no question that elimination of this incentive would have a drastic effect on charitable giving."[2]

And Jack Herman, who raises a lot of money as director of development at New York's Hospital for Joint Diseases and Medical Center, pointed out that the planning act is another obstacle to giving. "That has really slowed us down," he said. "Let's say a donor makes up his mind that he wants to contribute funds for a certain expensive piece of equipment, which would require health systems agency approval. Assuming the hospital believes such equipment is needed, the donor is put on hold while the hospital seeks approval. If approval is not given, the donor may shift the contribution elsewhere."[3]

Under the circumstances, it is astonishing that people like

Herman, Clarke, and others in the fund-raising and development field don't all quit their jobs and take up something with more promise for the future. Instead, they are optimistic. "Philanthropy is not drying up," said Herman. "Not in the least. There's plenty of money, just waiting to be donated to the right cause." A colleague who is eyeball-to-eyeball with the enemy, Brewster Terry of the Washington Hospital Center, sounds the same note. With the diminishing need for new hospital construction, Terry said, the emphasis today is on repair and renovation. "It will be harder to raise money," he explained, "but I still believe the satisfied patient, with the right encouragement, will be able to fill the hospitals' needs. There's plenty of money around." Terry thinks the physician is the key to fund raising. "The patient-doctor relationship is the crux," he said. "Our most important source of giving is the satisfied patient. The public doesn't care about how many meals were served last year or what our laundry bill was. They care about good patient care, and they want their donations used for patient care."[4]

If Terry and Herman are right, the outlook for hospital philanthropy may not be as devastating as it has seemed to the many hospital executives and trustees and others who have considered that it is dying and will eventually disappear, and who have consequently given up or made only half-hearted efforts to raise money for their hospitals—a tactic that is practically guaranteed to make their gloomy predictions true for their institutions. But even the cheerless allow that there will always be hospitals, though they are changing and may change more, so there will always be patient care. And the more persuasive argument is that there will always be philanthropy, the love of mankind that has existed for thousands of years and is not going to vanish, under whatever pressures, though it too may change with the changing society. Furthermore, it seems likely, if not inevitable, that there will always be Terrys and Hermans and Clarkes to direct some of the love, and some of the money, toward the institutions and causes they represent. They haven't always been recognized as such, but there have been fund raisers and development people around at least since the time of John the Baptist, and they are not likely to become extinct. So there will be hospital philanthropy, and the relevant questions are how much and what kind.

How much philanthropy for hospitals there is going to be depends first on how much money people will have to give and how much they will be disposed, and allowed, to give hospitals. These amounts obviously will be determined in part, and perhaps in large part, by the course of legislation and regulatory action in the Congress and in the states. Nobody knows what that will be, and speculation about the details is mostly a waste of time, but there are trends that people with hospital financing responsibilities can hardly afford to ignore. Thus over most of the past 20 years there has been a movement to legislate social programs on a national scale—most visible in the Great Society enactments of the 1960s but apparent also in the Kerr-Mills Act of 1961, in legislation liberalizing welfare and social security benefits, and in the Medicare amendments adding medical benefits for the disabled and those with endstage renal disease. .

In the latter half of this period, however, there has also been a countervailing trend arising from concern about the cost of these programs, and as a result we have had such measures as the Social Security Amendments of 1972 creating professional standards review organizations and the Section 1122 curbs on hospital expansion. Shortly afterward came the National Health Planning and Resources Development Act of 1974, establishing the health systems agencies, only a few of whose statutory functions and objectives have been implemented. In the past year or two the concern about costs has been heightened, and, while there have been few changes in the laws, regulatory interpretations and requirements in the federal spending programs have been tightened considerably. During most of this same period, too, in spite of continued strong efforts by liberal elements in the Congress, the labor movement, and the population, there has been a notable lack of action to add new entitlements. Instead of more social legislation, we have had Proposition 13 and other indications of disenchantment with taxes that are seen as burdensome, as well as preoccupation with the threatening energy shortage that most economists in late 1979 feared might bring on deep recession, if not depression, in the years just ahead.

So the long-term trend toward acceptance of more and more

social responsibility by government had been modified, and perhaps arrested, for the time being. But it was doubtful that it had been reversed. Even in the face of the threatened economic slowdown, the Congress was giving more serious consideration than it had in years to national health insurance proposals. An attempt to link national health insurance with a cost containment bill, which seemed illogical on the face of it, was evidence of the pervasive strength of the view that adequate health care for the whole population is an obligation of the government. It seemed likely that only a limited entitlement for protection against the expense of catastrophic illness or injury could be enacted in the near term, but it was apparent that the forces of social reform wouldn't go away, or would be back again if they did, perhaps quickly if recession deepened into depression, with massive unemployment, loss of health insurance coverage, and resulting hardship. In any event, some further limitations on the scope of philanthropy for hospitals might readily follow if even a limited form of health insurance were to be enacted.

The same forces can be expected to exert the same influences on tax legislation, with the same result. It was encouraging to hospitals and their fund raisers that a presidential proposal to extend the standard income tax deduction to millions of taxpayers was tossed out by a congressional committee without serious consideration, while a counterproposal that would give all taxpayers the opportuntiy to make a separate charitable deduction was introduced with promised support. But nothing of the sort happened, and the Filer Commission's recommendations for added tax incentives to giving didn't get anywhere either. It looked as though any tax legislation for the near term would be aimed at propping up sagging profits and employment, not at making giving easier for the wealthy.

A limited number of members of Congress may agree that the loss of support for hospitals that would follow any further restrictions on charitable giving would result in loss of services that would then have to be supplied by the government programs and would cost government more than the added tax revenues. And some lawmakers obviously believe the reverse—that the added tax revenues would outweigh the loss to hospitals, which they think has been exaggerated. But the majority probably consider that the more urgent problems of recession, inflation, and energy are all-consuming, and they won't feel constrained to make any decisions one way or the other about tax incentives for philanthropy. If there is plenty of money around, as Terry and Herman think there will be (and some fund raisers like Jerold Panas of San Francisco think tax incentives don't make much difference anyway),* how much of it are hospitals going to get, and what for?

There are some reasons to consider that the hospital share may diminish in the future. One reason is simply that some hospitals have quit trying, and the rule that you don't get money without asking for it isn't going to be suspended in the years ahead. Another reason is that all the headlines and broadcasts and conversations about Medicare and Medicaid and national health insurance help to spread the notion that the government is paying for health care for practically everybody and there is no real need for donations to help the sick poor, which in the past has been the strong core of the hospital appeal for philanthropic gifts. Still another reason is that hospitals might fail in the attempt to prevent government from using unrestricted gifts as an offset against Medicare and Medicaid payments, and donors would find other outlets for their contributions rather than see them appropriated to subsidized government programs. Finally, it is considered that widely publicized exposés about fund-raising frauds that raise millions for apparently worthy causes but use most of the money to enrich the promoters may have a dampening effect on giving to all charities but could hurt hospitals and health care most because some of the more flagrant abuses have been for "causes" related to health.

---

*In Des Moines, Iowa, one of the five U.S. cities whose "anatomy of giving" was the subject of intensive study by the Filer Commission, a local philanthropist had an altogether different view. "You have to realize that everyone is in a foundation because we have to be," Owen Fleming, a meat packing magnate, told a commission investigator. "You funnel great chunks of your money into a tax-exempt foundation, so you're expected to give part of it away, but you give it away the way you want to. The tiny percent you give away hardly matters. Anybody who says they'd give away the kind of money they do without a tax write-off is lying."[5]

These are all valid observations, and the effects could add up to a damaging loss of support for hospitals. But there are balancing circumstances suggesting that the hospital share of philanthropic beneficence may grow instead of shrinking. For every hospital that has quit trying to raise money, there may be a dozen that have intensified their efforts. As we have seen, the number of fund-raising hospital foundations has been increasing rapidly in the past two or three years. The motivation may have been not so much to increase the number and size of contributions as to get inside the stockade before the Indians attack, but the result has been more people spending more time asking, which is the best way in the world to ensure more giving. Moreover, the hospital effort is improving in quality as well as quantity. In place of the 10-week, hit-and-run campaigns for building funds that characterized most hospital fund raising for so many years, more and more institutions are making development a high-priority management responsibility and establishing departments headed by experienced executives who take part in the institutional planning and public relations programs and direct the continuing fund-raising enterprise. Some idea of the rate at which these activities have been accelerating is evident in the growth of the National Association for Hospital Development, which was organized in 1967 and had its offices in the secretary's briefcase and its meetings in hotel bedrooms until four or five years ago. Today it has a Washington headquarters office and staff, more than 1,000 members, and an education program aimed at keeping the membership informed about effective fund-raising techniques as well as legislative and regulatory developments affecting philanthropy and hospitals.

Although the government programs may have created a general impression that the sick poor are well provided for, there can't be many prospective donors who don't know, first, that there are millions of American men, women, and children who are left unprotected because of gaps and inadequacies in Medicare, Medicaid, and insurance coverage, which means there are hundreds in every hospital community, and second, that government payments don't by any means cover all the costs hospitals incur in caring for these patients, and they must either overcharge those who do pay or count on contributions, or both, to make up the difference. So the core appeal for donations to help the sick poor and near poor is still viable, and because charity, like the hospital, is largely a local phenomenon, it isn't difficult to demonstrate the truth to prospective donors. Furthermore, there are many needs and appeals—and more all the time—that are unrelated to the immediate needs of the sick poor, though few in any hospital that are unrelated to patient care. Unrestricted gifts are still important to hospitals, though it is likely for many reasons that the trend to donations earmarked by donors for specific purposes will continue. And while it isn't possible to forecast what will happen as the public funding agencies look greedily at unrestricted donations to hospital operating funds, and the AICPA decides what to do about reporting them, the hospital has some powerful allies helping to get this issue, and others, favorably resolved.

The Coalition of National Voluntary Organizations, which was founded several years ago to improve the climate for giving through research and public education on tax and other legislation, has recently joined the National Council on Philanthropy, an organization of foundations and other grant-making agencies, to form an umbrella group bringing donors and recipients together to work for the protection of private giving for public purposes. The new group, according to an announcement released at the time it was formed, will "attempt to foster a greater public understanding of the problems facing charitable organizations. Its basic goal will be to insure the survival of responsibly managed charitable institutions serving communities."

Among other goals, the new, enlarged coalition may be expected to help spread the word about charitable institutions and organizations that are not responsibly managed and are charitable to nobody but themselves. The phony organizations and cults that appeal to gullible and lost souls with messages of salvation may mulct their unsuspecting victims of millions, but sooner or later their schemes collapse, and it is unlikely that great sums are lost to legitimate charitable institutions because of them. The more insidious frauds are the respectable and worthy causes and institutions that are themselves victimized by promoters who keep or spend all but a token amount of the money they raise. The school or orphanage or church or hospital, and the donors, may remain unaware that they are being fleeced, sometimes year after year by repetition of the same scam, and the operators are usually careful to remain within the law.

State and federal authorities are aware of the threat and have been seeking to develop legislation and enforcement capabilities that will protect deserving institutions and causes, but it isn't easy always to distinguish between legitimate but justifiably expensive fund-raising methods, as for a new institution working with new lists of prospective donors, for example, and money-making schemes in disguise. The development and fund-raising associations have been working on the problem, and the new coalition may help to find a solution. Meanwhile, the only safe course for hospital trustees and executives is to make a thorough investigation of the credentials and references of any proposed fund-raising organization or consultant offering such services, to pay only fees agreed on in advance of the program and not based on a percentage of the funds raised, and to insist on auditing all statements of fund-raising expense. There will always be trimmers and swindlers in the fund-raising business, as there are in most others, but they haven't made much of a dent in real philanthropy in the past, and it doesn't seem possible that they will in the future.

There are sure to be changes in the nature of hospital philanthropy, however, because there are going to be changes in the nature of hospitals, and the best way to tell what philanthropy will look like is to see what hospitals will look like. Guesswork about the hospital of the future is a favorite pastime among hospital administrators and trustees and a staple topic for presentations at hospital meetings, and, of course, estimates vary all over the lot. The communications technologists tell us, for example, that the new, inexpensive, microminiaturized computers, combined with the new video image technology providing two-way coast-to-coast linkages, will make it possible within a short time for telemedical consultations to be conducted routinely by specialists in New York or Boston or Los Angeles for patients in New Mexico or Alaska, practically on demand, so it won't be necessary for hospitals outside the major population centers to have much more than beds and bedpans. The same technologists say their systems will permit simultaneous sharing of administrative services by hundreds, instead of a half dozen, hospitals. Laboratory, radiological, cardiological, and other medical data can be processed, perhaps for the whole country, in a handful of centers—not to mention the possibility that the same technology will permit many if not most of the diagnostic and therapeutic procedures now conducted in hospitals to be done in patients' homes, where other computer-managed devices will be doing everything but putting the children to bed.

Will any of this, or anything like it, actually be done? Probably some of it will be; in fact, some of it already is being done. But these visions of the future collide head-on with two powerful forces in our culture: local pride and local autonomy, and the personal component in medical care. The first suggests that technology will be accepted and used where it satisfies local pride and supports local autonomy and resisted or rejected where it doesn't; the second, the doctor-patient relationship, may be fragmented and attenuated by the technology, as it has been already, but it will not disappear. If anything, the philanthropist in a small town in, say, North Dakota, far from having to find other uses for his benevolence because the patients are all videophoning their symptoms and getting their treatments from specialists in Minneapolis, as the planning laws and the HSAs would like to see it done, may find new opportunities to help bring the new technologies to the local hospital and its doctors so their patients can be hospitalized at home and only the very sickest will have to be taken to the superspecialists in Minneapolis. Five years' experience with the planning law indicates that there are limits to the regionalization of medical care—a concept that has been around ever since Aesculapius planned his temples of healing for the islands of Cos, Epidaurus, and Cnidus in ancient Greece. Where it has been a case of doctors and patients on one side and planners on the other, it's no contest. The doctors and patients have had their way 90 percent of the time. There have been and will continue to be compromises where technology and local autonomy collide, but the community hospital and its values, including philanthropy, will survive, and the technology will do more to strengthen them than to weaken them.

The play of these forces has been at work for some time now, and the pattern events are taking is clear: The growth of multi-institutional systems is one of the outstanding developments in the hospital field in the past decade, with an estimated 40 percent of all acute general hospital beds in the country now in institutions affiliated with such systems, and the likelihood that as many as 75 percent of hospitals will be affiliated within a few years. There are all kinds of systems, ranging from arrangements to share plans and a few administrative services such as purchasing and data processing all the way to common ownership. And there are all sizes of systems, from two or three hospitals in the same area to a hundred or more in groups having units all over the country, as in some of the church systems and corporate chains.

This variety wasn't exactly what the planners had in mind, but it accomplished some, at least, of the planning goals of efficiency without sacrificing all the values of local pride, local autonomy, and local money. And it doesn't appear to have affected fund raising or giving one way or the other. Hospitals in the same city or town can share laundry and data processing services and still compete for donor interest, as they have always done, and the trustees who decide to join a management group to add resources and improve efficiency can carry on their fund-raising activities as before, perhaps more effectively if the pooled management includes experienced public relations and development talent, as many of them do. A donor in Colorado may be shy about making a donation to a hospital there if he thinks the beneficiaries are going to be not so much Colorado patients as Tennessee owners, but this is a problem any reasonably bright trustee or administrator or development officer can readily solve without losing a dollar of donations.

Another thing most of the forecasters agree on is that there will be less emphasis on beds and more on ambulatory services, at least for the short term. Planners and regulators and lawmakers are convinced that the hospital field is overexpanded, and they are determined not only to disapprove projects involving the addition of beds, except in the relatively few areas that are obviously underserved, but actually to shrink the system, as they like to say—a goal that is accomplished only rarely by actually closing down a hospital or service. To the extent that the supply of beds has been diminished, which isn't much, it is the result of trade-offs: We'll approve your replacement and modernization project, but only if the total number of beds when the project is completed is less than it was to begin with. The method is always aggravating and sometimes painful, and the shrinkage that results doesn't either help much or hurt much in the aggregate. But it is apparent that hospitals aren't going to be closed by executive order. As health economist Eli Ginzberg has said, "We don't know how to close hospitals, and neither do the British, or the Russians, or anybody else."[6] In the few areas where it has been tried here, the public uproar has been intimidating, and the planners have backed off. A few hospitals have died of natural causes, usually chronic underfinancing. Most of these were in poor areas or neighborhoods where they were badly needed but couldn't be supported, so the closings have simply added to the burdens of other institutions, without accomplishing any useful purpose, except for those who keep score only by bed count and think less is more.

Old-time development and fund-raising people look back nostalgically to the days when hospitals were expanding all over the place and as soon as one new building was completed and occupied, hospitals started planning, and raising money, for the next one. The addition that was needed because there simply wasn't room to take care of all the patients was comparatively easy to raise money for. The needs were plain to see and didn't take much explaining, the buildings and wings and floors could all be designated as memorials to the big givers, and the opportunities for gratifying every contributor's desire to be remembered were abundant. There are still hospitals that are engaged most of the time in building projects of one kind or another, and all except the newest ones have, and will continue to have, modernization needs. As Brewster Terry pointed out, it's harder to raise money for replacement and modernization, but it is being done every day, and as hospital functions change, new philanthropic opportunities will replace those that are thought to be lost because the number of beds stays the same or goes down.

The new emphasis on ambulatory services is one such opportunity. Hospitals are expanding outpatient departments, establishing outpatient surgical services, organizing and staffing neighborhood clinics and home care services, and reaching into their communities with programs of health education and promotion. Not all hospitals are doing all these things, obviously, and many aren't doing any of them. But more and more hospital people are coming to understand that with the pressures to hold down the number of beds and keep costs under control, these are going to be the principal areas of growth for the future. There are still a lot of hospital administrators and trustees who consider that proposals for neighborhood clinics and home care programs are impractical, and possibly insane. "We've got trouble enough keeping what we already have," they say. An increasing number, however, are beginning to realize that an extension of service is not just an added burden but a means of helping them keep what they have. Most of these new services can be self-sustaining in time, but they require some investment at the outset, and in most communities there will be donors who can be persuaded that these are special opportunities to bring needed care to the patients they want to help, extend service to their communities, and help ensure the growth and vitality of their hospitals. A number of hospitals, too, have sought and obtained support for the new services from foundations, many of which are more interested in innovative projects then they are in well-established, traditional institutions and services.

The whole field of preventive medicine, patient education, and public education about health, especially, is one that is just opening up for hospitals. In the past year or two, interest in it has grown so rapidly that the American Hospital Association has initiated a Center for Health Promotion to inform and assist hospitals that want to get such programs started. Hospitals doing this are taking part—and it should be a leading part—in an activity that began several years ago and is now gathering momentum and taking on the dimensions of a national movement involving government, industry, the health professions, and the public. This is the whole complex of interest and action growing out of the realization that we can keep on pouring more and more billions of dollars into biomedical research and medical treatment of illness and injury without greatly improving the health status of the population unless we also add something to the effort—heretofore relatively feeble—to prevent disease and injury, eliminate or modify environmental and social and behavioral causes of ill health, motivate people to take a greater share of responsibility for their own health, and teach them how.

In the past, interest in this approach has been limited to physicians and others in public health departments and a small number in public health and biomedical research and clinical medicine. The new surge of concern on the part of the federal administration and the Congress, industry, health insurers, and others was unquestionably sparked by the soaring cost of medical care in the government programs and, for industry, the cost of health insurance for employees and their families.

In government, a new Bureau of Health Education is conducting and contracting for studies designed to develop more precise knowledge about the methods that change behavior related to health, and to measure what health education programs accomplish. And a newer Office of Health Information, Health Promotion, Physical Fitness, and Sports Medicine is seeking to work with communities and states in their health promotion activities and also to establish policies and coordinate the many health education and physical fitness functions of government to provide cohesiveness for the total effort—an uphill task, judging from the label given the office, which is known as OHIHPPFSM. "The economic returns to prevention programs, including health education and health promotion programs, can be quite vast," said J. Michael McGinnis, M.D., deputy assistant secretary of the Department of Health, Education, and Welfare in charge of prevention and health promotion activities. "As we are able to develop a better understanding, not only on our own but on the part of other decision makers within the Administration, within the executive branch, and within the Congress, I think there will be a growing interest in these activities."[7]

There is indeed a growing interest in anything that will save money, and it is a basic assumption of the health promotion movement that healthier people will require less medical care, and it will cost less to make or keep them healthy than it does to take care of them when they aren't. The proposition for the most part is unproved, but industry, which is supposed to be steely-eyed and bottom-line minded, isn't waiting around for data; industry is going ahead on a broad front with programs of fitness, education, and promotion. Companies like IBM, American Telephone and Telegraph, Mobil, Cannon Mills, and others have initiated health promotion programs of various kinds. In some locations, for example, General Motors and Sears have subscribed to a health maintenance service that conducts broad workplace health education programs for all employees and workplace screening of some groups to identify poor health risks and initiate interventions such as exercise regimens, nutrition and stop-smoking classes; counseling for such problems as hypertension, obesity, and alcoholism; and medical referral or treatment for those with actionable symptoms.

The extent and cost of these programs varies according to the management's perception of the need and the benefit to be gained. There are no conclusive cost-benefit data as yet to demonstrate the payoff, but at one large corporation the initial screening identified a dozen cases of early neoplasms that were treated at an average cost of $2,000. Company physicians estimated the probable cost if the conditions had gone unrecognized and treatment had been delayed might have been in the neighborhood of $20,000 for each case, not to mention the suffering, lost time, and possible loss of life that might have occurred. This instance may have been unusual, but nearly all employers who have undertaken fitness, prevention, or health education programs for employees have reported improvements in absenteeism, productivity, and employee morale.

Although some services of this kind for industry have been organized and offered by foundations, health maintenance organizations, Blue Cross and Blue Shield Plans, and insurance companies, hospitals are a logical source, and in many communities the only source, of the information and personnel required. Many hospitals are already offering screening and counseling services for corporate executives, but most of the hospital prevention and health promotion programs that have been undertaken so far have been based at the hospitals and have had hospital patients and employees and community groups, rather than employed groups in industry, as their focus. But in any case, the field is wide open for development by hospitals—and for exploration with private foundations and donors who might be persuaded to provide startup funds.

According to a recent insurance company survey, the American people generally are skeptical about the reliability of health information handed out by public agencies, insurance companies, and their own employers, but they believe and trust the information they get from their doctors. Unfortunately, they don't get much. Seventy percent of the respondents said they felt their own doctor or doctors would be "very reliable sources of information about health and medical care," but only 47 percent were satisfied that they were getting all the information they needed. "The high regard most people have for their doctors and the high public trust in their opinions and expertise could be applied, to a far greater extent than has been done in the past, to change the diet habits and life-styles of most Americans," the survey report said.[8]

Changing diet habits and life-styles isn't easy, but with 60 percent of Americans overweight, 25 million with hypertension, and 16 percent of all families having a member with an acknowledged drinking problem, changing diets and life-styles may be the best chance we have to improve the nation's health, and philanthropists with any interest in health or education would have to consider that a well-organized health education program would do as much for the health of the community, and relieve as much suffering, as, say, a new children's wing or heart surgery. The hard part may be getting hospital trustees, administrators, physicians, and development people to consider that health education is just as much their job as sick children or heart patients are. Some will and some won't, and whether the hospital remains, as it has been, the central focus of all health care activities for its community or becomes just one of many agencies and institutions concerned with health depends as much as anything on how trustees and administrators and physicians—and donors—think about their roles.

One of the things they all have to be thinking about today is the challenge to hospitals posed by influential critics in government, in the universities, in industry, and in the professions who are convinced that the only alternative to the relentless rise of government regulation as a means of controlling the cost of medical and hospital care is the kind of change that will increase competition and give buyers—government, industry, health insurers, and consumers—a choice among alternative methods of seeking and receiving services. As a practical matter, this means increasing the reach and number of health maintenance organizations like the Kaiser Foundation Health Plans so that not just a few employers and groups and individuals in California, Minnesota, New York, and a few other places, but everybody, will have a valid choice between the services, and prices, of these prepaid group practices and those of the traditional fee-for-service practice of physicians with hospitalization insured by Blue Cross and Blue Shield and insurance companies. When this choice is ensured, the critics argue, the market for medical services will function more as other markets do to keep prices down.

The argument is supported by many well-documented studies showing that in comparable population groups fewer hospital days are used by HMO members than by those in traditional insured groups, a circumstance attributed to the fact that HMO doctors are paid fixed amounts to furnish comprehensive service for group members and thus have incentives to keep them out of hospitals, where costs are highest, whereas in fee-for-service practice the incentive is to admit patients to hospitals to ensure insurance coverage and "spend more and get more," as the critics say, overlooking many constraints in the existing system but making a persuasive case nevertheless for attempts to strengthen market forces in the medical economy.

Experience suggests that it might not work exactly the way the critics suppose. The Kaiser plans have been around for 40 years, and there were HMO-type groups long before Kaiser, and there have been many since then. Yet the total enrollment in HMOs today is less than 8 million, while Blue Cross, Blue Shield, and insurance companies have enrolled 180 million members over approximately the same period, for the obvious reason that this has been the way most doctors want to practice, and most insured groups and individuals are well satisfied with the way the system works and can see no particular reason to change.

But the virulent rise in costs of recent years has brought about an insistent demand for reforms in the system, and the increasingly severe grasp of regulation has a lot of hospital people and physicians thinking there must be a better way than this. The result has been a general agreement that some combination of regulation and the freer play of market forces would be preferable to more and more stringent rules and restrictions. A powerful group of management and labor leaders has recommended that corporations should encourage and even finance HMOs and offer to help them with technical and management expertise, which except for Kaiser hasn't been notably present in HMO development up to now. Legislative proposals that would seek to equalize the availability of HMOs and existing health insurance plans for employed groups have found some supporters in both the Senate and the House of Representatives, and some hospital boards have urged their doctors to organize groups and offer their services on a prepaid basis. There has been a feeling that if HMOs are to become a pervasive mode for the organization and financing of medical care, the hospitals had better have a part in their development.

All this costs money, and some observers see the support of such experiments in the delivery and financing of health care as an appropriate, and even necessary, function of private philanthropy. "In view of the critical role that the health care financing system plays in determining who receives health care, what kinds of services are provided, and at what price, the almost total absence of private foundation activity in the financing system area is noteworthy," said the report on private foundation expenditures of the Georgetown University Health Policy Research Group. "Today, the private insurers and private employers who pay a large part of the health care bill are much in the mood for experimenting with changes in their current practices. In this setting there may be a role for foundations to play, one which has not yet been widely exercised. With relatively small dollar outlays, foundations can stimulate reform by providing the planning grants needed to underwrite experiments and demonstrations affecting the financing system. They can also help support the evaluation of such experiments. This activity is essential to the documentation of the projects' impact on the delivery system, and for the dissemination of these findings to the financers and health care providers who set reimbursement policies."⁹

It might seem to be remote to the interest of individual donors who envision their beneficences saving lives and easing pains, but there may be some who can see past the bedside to the processes that get patients into the beds, and it's possible that easing the processes may be more socially useful than easing the pains.

Another informed observer mentions the same need for philanthropic support for experimentation in the financing system, and goes a step further. Commenting on health philanthropy for the future, Robert J. Blendon, M.D., of the Robert Wood Johnson Foundation said that "with basic health services more fully insured, the need for private philanthropy to provide venture capital for new types of health activities will substantially increase," and there will be a growing need to have an independent source of funds for experiments in the areas of research, education, and health service delivery. Government relies heavily on established interest groups and is slow to invest in new ideas, Blendon noted. "Thus many worthwhile concepts will never see the light of day unless substantial amounts of private giving can be made available for the planning and testing of new ideas." And because of cost problems, government will be prevented from moving aggressively to update standards of medical care, and, as a result, "a very special role will be created for private philanthropy in pursuit of qualitative goals in health."¹⁰

Finally, Blendon sees philanthropy as a guardian of the public interest: "Philanthropic health organizations, because of their financial independence from the government, can serve as the ombudsman for the public by supporting studies and special commissions to examine how well the public sector programs are meeting national objectives and how their performance might be improved," he concluded. But private philanthropy has become a relatively scarce national resource, he warned. "The pressing need to alter the current tax structure to achieve more equity in society has led some to propose that the incentives that encourage private gifts to philanthropic organizations be sharply reduced or totally eliminated. As time goes by, Americans will have to make a decision on how important a priority they place on maintaining pluralism in funding sources in fields such as health. This choice I suspect will be heavily influenced by the public's perception of the critical nature of the philanthropic contribution in the years ahead.''

An element that could help to tip the balance in favor of philanthropy would be a dramatic improvement in corporate giving, which the Filer Commission called "the last major undeveloped frontier" in philanthropy. One city whose business community has set an example for the rest of the country is Minneapolis, where 33 leading companies are giving 5 percent of their pre-tax income to charitable causes, led by the Dayton-Hudson Corporation, which has been doing it for 30 years—not just to help Minneapolis hospitals, colleges, museums, and other charities, according to Kenneth N. Dayton, chairman of the huge retail chain, but to keep the society free. "We believe there's only one reason for business," he said, "and that's to serve society. And if society doesn't perceive that business is doing it, it won't tolerate business. A certain amount of its efforts, its energies, and its resources must be devoted to building better environments in this nation. If not, the free enterprise system has a limited life span.''[11]

It isn't just business, but all givers and all providers of service who need to understand the critical role of philanthropy in the protection and preservation of freedom. "The sources of philanthropic giving or philanthropic involvement are very much the same sources that are conducive to economic development in this country, to free enterprise," Stanford sociologist Seymour Martin Lipsett told a conference on capital financing for hospitals. "These two go together, and insofar as philanthropy has declined I think the sources for its decline are also relevant to the decline of capitalism and free enterprise.''[12]

If the decline is to be arrested, the support must be strengthened all along the line. That's what philanthropists like Foster McGaw of Evanston, Illinois, and William Black of New York, and Malcolm Coutts of San Diego, and Webb Roberts of Dallas, and many others, have understood, and, as they have said, that has been one of the reasons for their generous gifts to voluntary hospitals and medical centers.

A recent visitor to the United States has an eloquent exegesis: "There was this ideal, still I think the most hopeful and important ideal that there is in the world, and it rested on the democratic organization of free men and it depended on something particular about the character of those men," William Rees-Moog, for many years editor of the *London Times,* said at a Chamber of Commerce dinner in Salt Lake City.[13] "Freedom is not something which just happens to a community, nor is it something which is preserved by accident. It is not a privilege which is ever long retained by those who are idle, who lack responsibility, who lack self-discipline. Those who prefer state discipline to self-discipline lose their freedom in the end and usually before very long. How stands this ideal of the free society with free men depending upon their own self-discipline to maintain the responsibility which the community requires if it is to survive?

"It is still in existence. If it were not in existence we should not be here. But it is impossible to pretend that it exists with the same vigor and self-confidence as it did a generation, or two generations, ago. There are those who wish to erode it, who wish to make their attack upon it. There are those who do not share this ideal. But, I believe, more insidious are those who would in fact pay some sort of shrugging lip service to this ideal but are not remotely prepared to pay the price which it involves.

"I find coming here that there is running through your community the idea that self-disciplined people must take responsibility for community affairs and take that responsibility as free men. That, I believe, is the principle which gave your nation its greatness in the world and made it, perhaps, the most successful experiment in political society that the world has ever seen. When I am here I know that that spirit is still strong. Long may it remain so, and long may its enemies be confounded."

How long what remains of our freedom will survive is something that both askers and givers can help to determine.

REFERENCES

Chapter 1

1. Panas, J. Interview, San Francisco, Apr. 22, 1978.
2. Peterson, C. N. Address at annual meeting, National Association for Hospital Development, Boston, Oct. 11, 1977.
3. Powell, B. Personal communication, Mar. 6, 1978.
4. Woodrum, D. Interview, Morgantown, WV, May 5, 1978.
5. Black, W. Before you give away money. *The Presidents' Forum*. New York City: Presidents' Professional Association, Inc., 1964,
6. Whitaker, B. *The Foundations: An Anatomy of Philanthropy and Society*. London: Eyre Methuen, 1974.
7. Coutts, M. B. Dedication address at Donald N. Sharp Memorial Community Hospital, San Diego, Apr. 24, 1977.
8. McGaw, F. Interview, Lake Forest, IL, Oct. 13, 1977.
9. Heldt, E. Interview, Long Beach, CA, Apr. 24, 1978.
10. Kirstein, G. *Better Giving*. Boston: Houghton, Mifflin & Co., 1975.
11. *Chicago Sun-Times,* Nov. 17, 1977.
12. Black, op. cit. (note 5).
13. Goulden, J. *The Money Givers*. New York City: Random House, 1971.

Chapter 2

1. Arthur Andersen & Co. *Tax Economics of Charitable Giving,* 6th ed. Chicago: Arthur Andersen & Co., 1971.
2. Arthur Andersen & Co. *Tax Reform Act of 1976.* 2nd ed. rev.

Chicago: Arthur Andersen & Co., 1976.

3. Clarke, J. Draft memorandum on Voluntary Hospital-Medical Center Philanthropic Support Act, Jan. 17, 1979.

4. New England Association for Hospital Development. *Special Report to the Massachusetts Rate Setting Commission,* Feb. 1979.

5. Silverstein, L. Preface. In: *Research Papers Sponsored by the Commission on Private Philanthropy and Public Needs,* vol. 1. Washington, DC: U.S. Department of the Treasury, 1977, p. v.

6. The donee group: report and recommendations. In: *Research Papers Sponsored by the Commission on Private Philanthropy and Public Needs,* op. cit. (note 5), vol. 1, p. 49.

7. *Giving in America: Toward a Stronger Voluntary Sector.* Report of the Commission on Private Philanthropy and Public Needs. Introduction and Summary, Washington, DC: Department of the Treasury, 1977, p. 23.

8. The donee group: report and recommendations. In: *Research Papers Sponsored by the Commission on Private Philanthropy and Public Needs,* op. cit. (note 5), p. 59.

9. Morgan, J., and others. Results from two national surveys of philanthropic activity. In: *Research Papers Sponsored by the Commission on Private Philanthropy and Public Needs,* op. cit. (note 5), vol. 1, p. 160.

10. Ibid, p. 228.

11. Feldstein, M., and Taylor, A. The income tax and charitable contributions: estimates and simulations with the treasury tax file. In: *Research Papers Sponsored by the Commission on Private Philanthropy and Public Needs,* op. cit. (note 5), vol. 3, p. 1437.

12. Boskin, M., and Feldstein, M. Effects of the charitable deduction on contributions by low income and middle income households: evidence from the National Survey of Philanthropy. In: *Research Papers Sponsored by the Commission on Private Philanthropy and Public Needs,* op. cit. (note 5), vol. 3, p. 1450.

13. Boskin, M. Estate taxation and charitable bequests. In: *Research Papers Sponsored by the Commission on Private Philanthropy and Public Needs,* op. cit. (note 5), vol. 3, p. 1479.

14. *Giving in America,* op. cit. (note 7).
15. Ibid, p. 17.
16. Nelson, R. Private giving in the American economy. In: *Research Papers sponsored by the Commission on Private Philanthropy and Public Needs,* op. cit. (note 5), vol. 1, p. 129.
17. Blendon, R. The changing role of private philanthropy in health affairs. In: *Research Papers Sponsored by the Commission on Private Philanthropy and Public Needs,* op. cit. (note 5), vol. 2, p. 650.
18. American Hospital Association Survey. Reported in *Giving USA: 1977 Annual Report of the American Association of Fund-Raising Counsel, Inc.* New York City: AAFRC, 1977.
19. Chayet, N. Address at New England Hospital Assembly, Boston, Mar. 29, 1978.
20. Unger, W. Address at annual meeting, National Association for Hospital Development, Oct. 10, 1977.

Chapter 3

1. Goulden, op. cit. (chapter 1, note 13).
2. DeTocqueville, A. *Democracy in America.* New York City: Harper and Row, 1966 (originally published in 1845).
3. Schaff, P. *A Sketch of the Political, Social and Religious Character of the United States.* New York City: Charles Scribner, 1855.
4. Lipset, S. M. Comments on a paper presented at Conference on Capital Financing for Hospital Facilities, University of Pittsburgh, Nov. 20, 1976.
5. Packard, F. *Some Account of the Pennsylvania Hospital: From Its First Rise to the Beginning of the Year 1938.* Philadelphia: The Pennsylvania Hospital, 1938.
6. Ibid.
7. Bremner, R. Private philanthropy and public needs: historical perspective. In: *Research Papers Sponsored by the Commission on Private Philanthropy and Public Needs,* op. cit. (chapter 2, note 5), vol. 1, p. 92.
8. Ibid, p. 93.

Chapter 4

1. Gonser, Gerber, Tinker, Stuhr. *On Development* (compiled from the *Bulletin on Philanthropy and Development).* Chicago, GGTS, 1977.
2. Rimalover, J. Address at annual meeting, National Association for Hospital Development, Boston, Oct. 12, 1977.
3. Ziettlow, C. Personal communication, Feb. 1978.
4. Donovan, J. Address at annual meeting, National Association for Hospital Development, Boston, Oct. 10, 1977.

Chapter 5

1. Gonser, Gerber, Tinker, Stuhr, op. cit. (chapter 4, note 1).
2. Herman, J. Address at annual meeting, National Association for Hospital Development, Houston, Oct. 10, 1976.
3. Hobbie, W. Cultivate major donors by knowing when to ask. Paper presented at New England Association for Hospital Development, Newport, RI, Sept. 13, 1976.
4. Slosson, M. Interview, Los Angeles, Apr. 25, 1978.
5. Heldt, E. Interview, Long Beach, CA, Apr. 24, 1978.
6. Panas, J. Interview, San Francisco, Apr. 22, 1978.
7. Bonney, W. Address at annual meeting, National Association for Hospital Development, Boston, Oct. 10, 1977.
8. Mayo, T. Address at annual meeting, National Association for Hospital Development, Boston, Oct. 10, 1978.
9. Stuber, J. Managing a deferred giving program. Trusts and Estates. *Journal of Estate Planning and Administration,* Sept. 1977.
10. Hornor, T. Address at annual meeting, National Association for Hospital Development, Boston, Oct. 11, 1977.
11. Powell, B. Interview, Dallas, Mar. 1, 1978.

Chapter 6

1. Whitaker, op. cit. (chapter 1, note 6).
2. Haney, W. Interview, Boston, Oct. 10, 1977.
3. Schwartz, J. The role and selection of professional counsel. In: Roland, W., editor, *The Handbook of Institutional Advancement.* San Francisco: Jossey-Bass, 1977.
4. Harris, F., and Klepper, A. Corporate philanthropic public

service activities. Summarized in Commentary on Recommendations. In: *Research Papers Sponsored by the Commission on Private Philanthropy and Public Needs,* op. cit. (chapter 2, note 5), vol. 1, p. 43.

5. Detzel, D. Quoted in Gonser, Gerber, Tinker, Stuhr, *Bulletin on Public Relations and Development for Hospitals,* Apr. 1979.

Chapter 7

1. Foundations, private giving and public policy. In: *Research and Recommendations of the Commission on Foundations and Private Philanthropy.* Chicago: University of Chicago Press, 1970.
2. Nielson, W. *The Big Foundations: A Twentieth-Century Fund Study.* New York City: Columbia University Press, 1972.
3. Craig, J., and others. *Private Foundation Health Expenditures: A Summary Analysis.* Washington, DC: Health Policy Research Group, Georgetown University School of Medicine, Oct. 1978.
4. Vazquez, C. Address at annual meeting, National Association for Hospital Development, San Diego, Dec. 13, 1978.
5. Dunlap, H. Interview, Los Angeles, Apr. 25, 1978.
6. Vitello, J. Giving gets its own house. *Hospitals, J.A.H.A. 49:95, June 1, 1975.*
7. Regan, W. *Regan Report on Hospital Law,* Oct. 1974.
8. Vitello, J. Exposure draft threatens the future of the hospital foundation. *Hospitals, J.A.H.A.* 52:155, June 16, 1978.
9. American Institute of Certified Public Accountants, Subcommittee on Health Care Matters. Clarification of reporting practices concerning hospital-related organizations: proposed statement of position. New York City: AICPA, Aug. 31, 1979.
10. Whitney, J. Conserving hospital revenues by the use of foundations. Address at Ohio Association for Hospital Development, Columbus, Dec. 6, 1978.
11. Memel, S. Address at annual meeting, National Association for Hospital Development, San Diego, Dec. 13, 1978.

Chapter 8

1. Roper Organization, Inc. *Roper Reports,* July 1979.

2. Porte, B. Address at annual meeting, National Association for Hospital Development, San Francisco, Oct. 1974.

Chapter 9

1. Terenzio, J. Address at Conference on Capital Financing for Hospital Facilities, University of Pittsburgh, Nov. 20, 1976.
2. *American Medical News,* Jan. 12, 1979.
3. Ibid.
4. Ibid.
5. Kentfield, C. The anatomy of giving: private philanthropy in Des Moines. In: *Research Papers Sponsored by the Commission on Private Philanthropy and Public Needs,* op. cit. (chapter 2, note 5), vol. 2, p. 998.
6. Ginzberg, E. Comment in discussion, Conference on Capital Financing for Hospital Facilities, University of Pittsburgh, Nov. 20, 1976.
7. *Health Education Reports,* July 17, 1979.
8. *Health Maintenance.* Report of a survey conducted by Louis Harris & Associates for the Pacific Mutual Life Insurance Co., Nov. 1978.
9. Craig, J., and others, op. cit. (chapter 7, note 3).
10. Blendon, R. The changing role of private philanthropy in health affairs. *New Engl J Med,* May 1, 1975, p. 946.
11. *New York Times,* July 23, 1978.
12. Lipset, S. M. Address at Conference on Capital Financing for Hospital Facilities, University of Pittsburgh, Nov. 20, 1976.
13. *Deseret News,* Mar. 31, 1978.

INDEX